Wellness
Mind-Body
Activities

HOWARD D. BLAZEK

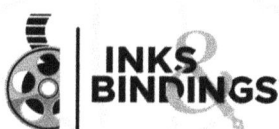

Copyright © 2024 by Howard D. Blazek

ISBN: 979-8-88615-225-8 (Paperback)
    979-8-88615-226-5 (Ebook)

All rights reserved. No part of this publication may be reproduced, distributed, or transmitted in any form or by any means, including photocopying, recording, or other electronic or mechanical methods, without the prior written permission of the publisher, except in the case brief quotations embodied in critical reviews and other noncommercial uses permitted by copyright law.

The views expressed in this book are solely those of the author and do not necessarily reflect the views of the publisher, and the publisher hereby disclaims any responsibility for them.

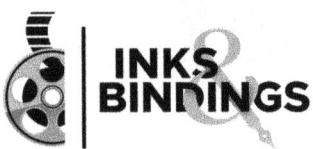

Inks and Bindings
888-290-5218
www.inksandbindings.com
orders@inksandbindings.com

The purpose of this book is to help you lessen any stress or physical pain you may have and to help you move toward Wellness.

No attempt is made to diagnose any illness or provide any type of medical advice. Please see your health care practitioner if you have questions or problems with your medical condition.

This book contains tips and techniques to use yoga, meditation and related activities. Check with your health care professional if you have any doubts about doing any of the activities in this book.

Be aware of your condition. Be well.

The author is responsible for the content of this book. It includes common Wellness knowledge, personal experience (yoga classes, training workshops, and lectures), the internet (online meditations and classes including videos, audios and emails) and input from his Kundalini collaborator.

Any errors, omissions, or mis-interpretations are the sole responsibility of the author.

Foreword

> Congratulations on finding this book. Bringing it to market has been an adventure.
>
> Originally published as *Wellness Activities & Insights* by Dreamer's Point in January of 2023, they disappeared just as they completed and printed it. Unable to contact them, I republished the book with Brilliant Books Literary in May of 2023. Less than a year later, they too were gone.
>
> This is the same book with a new title and formatting changes and corrections. Enjoy.

The purpose of this book is to help you be free of pain in your body and trouble in your mind. Hopefully, this information and these activities will help you continue on a journey to complete Wellness. Read. Enjoy. Do the activities that resonate with you. Ignore or skip the ones that do not interest you.

Late in high school, I had read an article that the hedonists of old (thought of as pleasure-seekers in the popular world) actually had a philosophy or goal of "no pain in the body and no trouble in the mind." I really liked that concept and it has stayed with me throughout the years. The activities and information in this book are dedicated to this goal. May you have:

- Less or no pain in your body
- Less or no trouble in your mind

The twin scourges of stress and inflammation affect almost everyone in today's world. Hopefully, the information and activities in this book will help you to relieve some of the physical, mental, or emotional stress you may have. Many of the activities will help you reduce any inflammation you may have in your brain or body.

Wellness has been defined as "the quality or state of being in good health" as well as "the process of learning about and engaging in behaviors that are likely to result in good health." Hopefully, the activities in this book will help you move toward wellness.

After high school I got caught up in the material world, eating and drinking too much, consumed by success and achievement. With life getting in the way, it was not until my mid-60s when I became totally serious about trying to be healthy, fit, and flexible. Yoga and meditation were the way. I would devote the remaining years of my life to becoming the best version of myself and to helping others.

As I worked to rejuvenate myself, I found that my stiff, aging body was betraying me and my thoughts kept falling into negative patterns, and my emotional life was insecure.

I began collecting "simple things." Simple ways to get better. Many are included here, together with my thoughts, ideas, and experiences.

Address any questions or comments about this book to me at howardblazek@gmail.com.

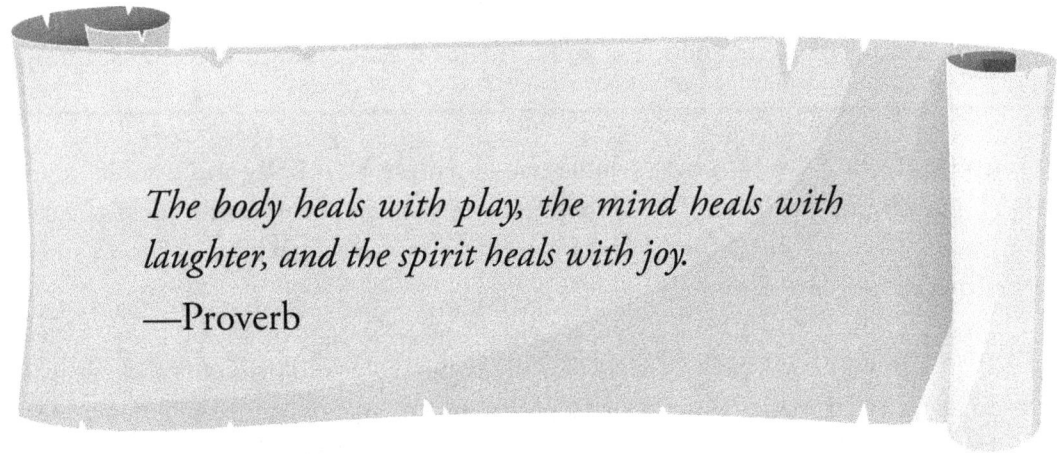

The body heals with play, the mind heals with laughter, and the spirit heals with joy.
—Proverb

Contents

Foreword v

Table of Contents vii

First Word xi

Getting Started 1

    Living in the Present 1

    21 Days 2

    General 2

    Going in Order 3

    Counting 3

    Scanning 3

    Contents 4

    Other 4

Energy 5

    Energy and Information 6

    Life Force 6

    Energy and Attention 7

    Chakras 8

    Meridians 8

    Acupuncture/Acupressure Points 9

    Energy Body 9

7 Major Chakras	*10*
Energy Centers	*11*
Summary	*12*

Self 13

Who Are You? What Do You Want?	*13*
You Are a Miracle	*15*
Preconceptions	*15*
Energy Being	*16*
Forgiveness	*17*
Summary	*21*

Thinking 23

Affirmations	*24*
Mirror Work	*25*
Intention, Inner Wisdom, Gratitude	*27*
Meditative State	*28*
Sample Affirmations	*28*
Visualization	*29*
Going Deeper	*29*
Contrast	*30*
Chakra Affirmations	*31*
Summary	*33*

Breathing 35

Mindfulness Exercise	*36*
Yoga and Breathing	*37*
Voluntary	*37*
Meditation and Breathing	*39*

    Pranayama & Alternative Nostril Breathing 43

    Summary 45

Meditation 47

    Purpose 47

    Classic Pose 51

    Meditating 51

    Mantras 53

    Meditative State 57

    Brain Waves 58

    Mindfulness 60

    Chakra Healing 66

    Energy Meditation 68

    Summary 70

Hands 71

    Warm-up Exercises 71

    3-Finger Technique 73

    Acupressure Points 73

    Mudras 75

    Restless Night 79

    Summary 81

Yoga-Related Activities 83

    Simple Is, Simple Does 83

    EFT (Emotional Freedom Technique) 86

    Walking 100

    Intestine Exercise 101

    Stretching 102

  Twist and Turn.. *110*

  Summary *114*

Yoga **115**

  Chair Yoga *116*

  Stress Relief—Lower Back and Hip Basics...................... *117*

  Upper Back Routine *120*

  Wake Up and Move in the Morning *122*

  Summary *128*

Sources and Additional Information **129**

  Getting Started *129*

  Energy *130*

  Self *131*

  Thinking.. *131*

  Breathing *132*

  Meditation *133*

  Hands *134*

  Yoga-Related Activities *134*

  Yoga... *135*

  Books *135*

  Web Sites *137*

Going Forward.. **139**

Acknowledgements **141**

First Word

These self-help tips and techniques are meant to help you understand and use yoga, meditation, and related activities for your own benefit and the benefit of others. They have brought me tremendous relief, joy, and hope. I hope they work for you.

Each of us is a miracle. I hope this book helps you understand just how precious you are. I hope you are interested in positive change (of your condition or situation) for yourself and others. There are no "should do's" or "must do's" in these pages; there is only "I can do it." Self-love and acceptance of self and others are essential for your personal growth.

My interest in yoga and meditation was re-ignited in my middle 60s. After struggling with a stiff, sluggish body, I began getting better. Today, I am healthier than I was 15 years ago. I have experienced so much wonder, love, and joy in the last few years that it no longer matters how old I am. I am glad to be me and have the opportunity to continue to learn and grow.

I have no desire to promote any religion, organization or belief system. I have referenced individuals who have produced some really nice work which may be helpful to you. Yoga can be thought of as a discipline or union (of mind, body, spirit). This book describes the energy body, chakras, and more. These concepts may be foreign to you. Use what makes sense to you. Have fun. This content may help you heal the trouble in your mind and pain in your body.

It's a different world now.

When I was growing up in the 1940s and 1950s in the Midwestern United States, Indian yogis were shown in cartoons as small and thin with a long white beard. They were usually wearing a turban. They were shown lying on a bed of nails or charming a snake out of a basket by playing a flute. Some were pictured living in a cave or sitting on the top of a mountain.

In 1970, I went to a presentation given by an Indian yogi. Oh my. What a challenge to my preconceptions. He was a tall, strong-shouldered, big-chested man with long, dark hair and a long, full dark beard. He emanated power and strength, and looked more like a pro football player than my stereotype of a yogi.

During a brief lecture, he put down drugs and alcohol. The hippies were shocked. As one woman cried out, "But drugs are what got us here." While the hippies sat in stunned silence, the non-hippie straights were more vocal as in, "But even our Lord, Jesus Christ, drank wine!"

I love his reply to this earnest Christian and still cherish it all of these years later, "No. This I do not believe. I do not believe a man so powerful he can raise the dead could also drink alcohol." I had, indeed, entered a different world.

After drifting off into school and work, leading a mundane life, I got caught up in yoga and meditation decades later when I was in my 60s. I answered an ad for a free checkup in connection with yoga classes. Surprisingly (shocking to me), it was difficult for me to lie flat on my back without pain. I knew I had gained weight, was stiff and not very flexible. I knew that arthritis was restricting my movements, but I had not realized the extent of my slowdown. I had gotten old and was only growing older. At the same time, the person checking my condition had me do some things with my feet (toe-tapping, foot rotations, and massage). It felt great. I was hooked. There was hope for me.

My journey started by doing yoga in order to be healthier and feel better. Simple exercises to help my body only opened me to increasing wonder. I would find that mind, body, and spirit are all interrelated. I would immerse myself in reading and religiously practice meditation (a life-long habit of mine which had fallen into disuse). I would find that I was filled with preconceptions that had brought me neither peace nor satisfaction. I would listen to my chattering, monkey mind and realize that many of my thoughts, especially those about myself were negative. I would learn that much of my stiffness and physical discomfort was the result of emotional residue held in my body from traumatic events that occurred long ago. I was on the road to wellness.

Slowly but surely, I discovered a world where I choose to be happy, healthy, abundant, grateful, and generous with my time and resources. My journey has not been without pitfalls and problems. It has been full of starts and stops with retention of negative habits and thought patterns. I still have not arrived, but I am really beginning to enjoy my arriving. As they say, "The journey is the destination." And what a journey it has been.

This collection of tips and techniques is a direct outgrowth of my experiences, input from friends and extensive study and reading. If anything in this book or the accompanying materials helps you to feel better, know more, be filled with hope or joy, or otherwise grow and prosper, I feel this work has been a worthwhile endeavor.

Please note that I am but an egg, an initiate or novice at best. The contents of this work are things I have learned in my attempts to heal myself and improve my state of being. They are not pronouncements from a knower but rather, hints from a seeker.

> Follow the wisdom of your body. You are a miracle. Treat yourself like one.

The journey of a thousand miles begins with one step.
—Lao-Tze

The only impossible journey is the one you never begin.
—Tony Robbins

Whether you think you can or you think you can't, you're right.
—Henry Ford

Getting Started

As with the Greek hedonists of old, the purpose of this collection of activities is to help you "relieve trouble in the mind and pain in the body." Going further, it is aimed at enabling you to help heal yourself and others, and to change your condition for the better. Scientists, medical doctors, alternative medicine advocates, and wellness coaches are all saying with an increasingly loud voice that the self-healing powers of each of us is much greater than previously thought. This book has the goal of providing activities for your personal growth and self-healing.

> Do <u>not</u> view anything in these pages as a substitute for professional care and support. Always listen to the wisdom of your body. Check with your medical providers if you have any question or doubts about doing any of the activities in this book. Do well. Be well.

Living in the Present

Meditation and yoga both require you to be in the present moment to be totally effective. Pay attention to what you are doing and experiencing now. Be present here and now.

As that great pundit, Kung Fu Panda, said in his first movie, "The past is history, the future is mystery, today is a gift which is why we call it the present." Many teachers point out that the present moment is all we have. Accept and cherish it.

While humans have this great gift of being able to remember the past and anticipate the future, they may ignore the present moment. Mindfulness, the art of paying attention to your inner and outer world NOW, would be the greatest gift I could give you, if it were mine to give.

Be here now. Stay present. Just be. Whatever words it takes, pay attention to the moment, especially when doing the activities in this book. The benefits of staying in the present will explode exponentially.

21 Days

Although the exact length of days and number of repetitions is open to debate, psychologists tell us that it takes several days of doing or not doing something to form a habit. If you can do something each day for 21 (or your golden number) days you build the necessary neural connections to be able to continue doing it on a daily basis. Kundalini yoga uses 40 days to change a habit.

The message is consistency. Be consistent over time.

As possible, stay with the activities in this book that resonate with you on a daily basis for as many days as it takes to feel you are doing something natural and helpful. For example, if you can replace negative chatter in your brain with positive affirmations for an extended period of time you will build up the necessary neural patterns to continue to have positive thoughts as second nature.

General

Do the exercises either barefoot or wearing nonslip socks or yoga slippers in order to connect to earth energy through the soles of your feet. Wear comfortable clothing that does not restrict your movements. Be sure to warm up before attempting to do anything strenuous.

According to Kundalini Yoga, we have 72,000 nerve endings in our feet which are receptive to subtle energies when uncovered. In order to receive the full energy produced by the exercises and movements, doing them with bare feet is ideal.

If you meditate or do simple yoga movements while sitting in a straight-backed chair, it is most effective to have bare feet that are flat on the ground for meditation and other activities.

Listen to the wisdom of your body. Use common sense. You know your body better than anyone else. The goal is to become fit and flexible. "No pain, no gain" is <u>not</u> appropriate.

Think "no pain, no pain." The activities in this book are designed to help you move, relax, and experience joy and wonder without stress or pain.

Going in Order

Jump around in this book. Although adequate breathing techniques are essential to both yoga and meditation, and some yoga movements build on earlier ones, the activities in this book do not have to be done in order. This is basically a free-form text that enables you to go to any section or part which appeals to you. Do what gets you interested and involved. You do not have to go through the book in order or do every activity.

Counting

Some of the simple repetitive exercises may require a large number of repetitions. For example, toe-tapping or bobbing up and down may be done hundreds of times depending on your purpose and condition. When counting, try it this way: 1, 2, 3, 4, 5, 6, 7, 8, 9, 10, 1, 2, 3, 4, 5, 6, 7, 8, 9, 20, etc. Counting will let you know how many you are doing and help you to stay in the present by giving you something to focus on.

If you are doing a large number of repetitions, you can also use a timer. Whether you count or use a timer, remain in the present and focus on what you are doing. Worrying about other tasks can wait until you are done meditating or exercising.

Scanning

Before starting and after finishing an exercise, it is a good idea to scan your body. How do you feel? You can start with your toes and work up to the crown of your head or work from your head to toes or just let yourself be drawn to a particular area of your body. As several of my teachers have said, "Awareness brings about change." Scanning to become aware of a physical condition is a good way to start becoming healthier. You do not have to actively change anything.

Over time it is hoped that you become increasingly tuned to your body and how it feels. As you become more adept at becoming aware of your condition you may feel healing taking place. Do not suppress or repress your feelings; cherish them and let them have a voice.

Contents

You may not be able to do all of the activities. Just do what you can and what you enjoy. Even if you have trouble with some of the physical exercises, you should be able to do affirmations, most of the breathing exercises, the hands activities and meditation.

Other

Have fun. Be joyful. If there is something you do not understand, it is probably due to my lack of clarity. Do not worry about it. Smile at my ineptitude and move on to something that is clear to you. There are no "should do" or "musts" in this book, only "may do," "can do," and "will do."

> *Energy cannot be created or destroyed; it can only be changed from one form to another.*
> —Albert Einstein
>
> *Everything is energy and that is all there is to it. Match the frequency of the reality you want and you cannot help but get that reality. It can be no other way. This is not philosophy. This is physics*
> —Albert Einstein

Energy

This entire book is about energy. When someone talks about energy, you may think of light, sound, and vibration, the three ways our senses perceive energy. You also know that there are all kinds of energy that you cannot see, hear, or touch, such as electricity and radio waves.

Going further, everything in the material universe is made up of energy. Matter, as you may have learned in physics class in high school, is ultimately energy. A very small amount of matter contains a very large amount of energy as shown by Einstein's equation $E=MC^2$ (the energy contained in matter is equal to the mass of an object times the speed of light squared which is a very large number indeed as the speed of light is 186,000 miles per second). Think of your solid physical body as ultimately consisting of energy in motion. On a larger scale, think of yourself as a bio-magnet living in a huge field of energy, who interacts with other bio-magnets. You are an energy field interacting with other energy fields operating within larger energy fields.

Look around you. Everything that you can see, hear, feel, or touch is energy constantly moving. If you had the eyes for it, that solid, immovable tree is really energy in motion.

Jean Huston (as quoted by Melissa Kruz) puts it this way:

The Universe is energy—the same energy that is the source of our being and everything there is.

In fact, the greatest scientific discovery of all time is indeed the realization modern Quantum Physics first uncovered in the early 20th century but which was long known in Eastern philosophies and native cultures—the fact that everything in the Universe is only this singular energy in a constant state of change.

Einstein said that matter is just slow energy that can be experienced by our senses.

What does this mean to you? Well, first of all, it's really good news. Forget appearances. You are an energy field. There are all kinds of yoga exercises, meditations, and related activities to bring fresh energy into your system, circulate it through your system, and release old, stagnant, or excessive energy that is no longer needed by you. You can become brighter, vibrate at a more harmonious frequency, rejuvenate the cells of your body and otherwise strengthen and help yourself.

James Ray, as quoted in *The Secret*, says:

"Most people define themselves by this finite body, but you're not a finite body. Even under a microscope you're an energy field."

Energy and Information

As we go smaller and smaller, getting into subatomic particles, quantum physicists tell us that basically everything is made up of the same stuff.

In the physical universe, there is basically energy and information. Information is what turns some energy into becoming a tree, some into a rock, and some into an animal or a human being. In other words, different patterns or configurations of energy become different things according to our senses.

Life Force

In addition to each of us being an energy field, there is a life force that permeates our bodies. In Asian traditions, it has been called Ki, chi, qi, life particles, and prana. The body is the vehicle for this life force.

The Hindu's emphasize prana, which means breath. The study of prana or breath is called pranayama, which is an incredibly detailed system of breathing techniques. For those of you who really get into breath work, I recommend studying pranayama or finding a teacher who is familiar with it. I use Ki, chi, and qi interchangeably with each referring to the energy or life force that flows through us. The term, life particles, is used by Ilchi Li, the founder of Dahn yoga, to identify the smallest possible particles that contain both information and life.

Much of yoga and meditation is based around being able to sense and be aware of the life force that flows through us. There are movements, postures and meditations to help us accumulate, circulate, and release energy.

This life force flows through you and forms your subtle body.

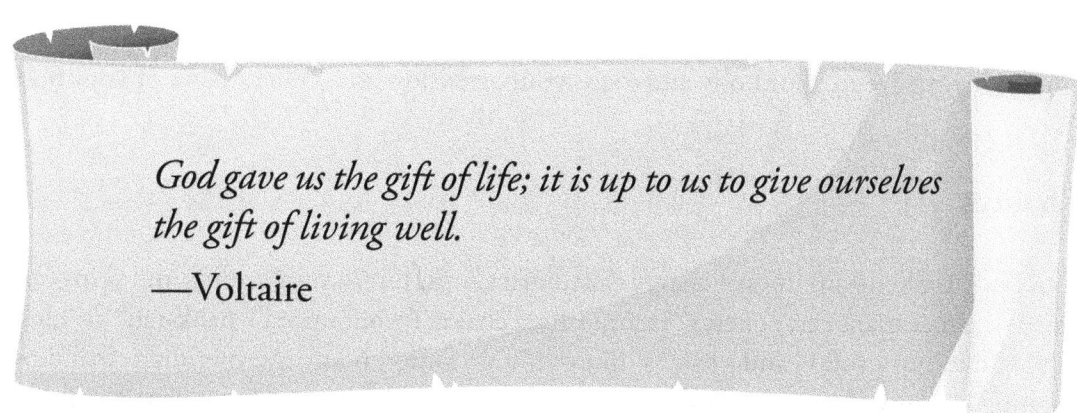

God gave us the gift of life; it is up to us to give ourselves the gift of living well.
—Voltaire

Energy and Attention

There are many ways to receive, circulate, and release the energy that flows through you. Some of these ways are included in the Hands, Meditation, Activity, and Yoga sections of this book.

Your energy goes where your attention goes.

Where is your attention right now? That is where your energy is going. This principle can be easily demonstrated:

- Sit quietly in a straight-backed chair with your spine straight and your feet flat on the ground
- Focus on one of your feet (either right or left is okay). Give all of your attention to this foot. Picture it. Visualize how it would look from the inside out. Pay attention to your toes, the sides, top, and bottom of your foot as well as the heel of this foot. How do the parts feel, look and connect with each other?
- Continue to focus on your foot for a minute or two, visualizing and becoming sensitive to each part of it
- Now, sit back, relax, and take a few deep breaths. How do your feet feel?

Is the foot you focused on warmer, tingly, or more energetic than your other foot? Most people report that their two feet now feel very different with more energy and sensation in the one on which they focused their attention.

Giving attention to an energy center or body part gives energy to that part. This is useful to know when you scan your body and focus your attention on different parts of your body.

Chakras

Your body is filled with lines of energy called meridians. Just as your arteries and veins carry blood, the meridians carry energy. Technically, a chakra (pronounced "shahk-rah" or "chuk-ruh"; C like S or a soft C and a soft "a" like the "a" in father) is any two meridians that cross, resulting in many chakras in your body. When people say "chakra" they are usually referring to one of the seven major chakras or energy centers in your body. These seven chakras are basically located along the spine with three lower chakras and three upper chakras mediated by the central heart chakra. Each chakra has distinct attributes and characteristics. They are energy centers with a large number of meridians passing through them.

1. Root chakra (located on the pericardium slightly below the base of the spine).
2. Sacral chakra (located on the spine about 2 inches below the navel).
3. Solar Plexus chakra (located above the navel and below the sternum).
4. Heart chakra (located in the center of the chest).
5. Throat chakra (located in the center of the throat).
6. Third eye (located on the forehead between the eyebrows slightly above the eyes.
7. Crown chakra (located on the very top of the head).

Chakras have been studied for thousands of years and are central to Hinduism, Buddhism, and other Eastern religions and philosophies. Although there are some differences of opinion regarding the origin, colors, characteristics, and other details regarding chakras, this does not concern us.

If these energy centers are closed or out of balance, it results in physical or mental discomfort.

Meridians

Our bodies are permeated by energy lines called meridians. There are 12-20 major meridians located in the body (the number varies by system, philosophy and definition) and many more minor ones. Think of chakras as bus terminals, the major meridians as super highways and the minor meridians as roads.

Just as there can be blockages in blood vessels that can cause us harm including stroke and heart disease, we can have blockages in our energy lines. Although more subtle, opening these blockages improves your health and well-being.

Acupuncture/Acupressure Points

There are hundreds of acupressure points along our meridians. These points can be cleared and/or activated by applying pressure (acupressure) on a point or by using small needles (acupuncture). You can remember the relationships between chakras, meridians, and acupressure points using a calendar:

1. Chakras (seven major chakras; same as the number of days in a week; act as a center or a kind of bus terminal for the energy lines (meridians) that run throughout your physical body).
2. Meridians (12-20 major meridians and many minor ones; loosely the same as the number of months; act as roads or lines of energy throughout the body).
3. Acupressure/acupuncture points (hundreds of points, approximately 365 or the number of days in a year; serve as bus stops along the meridian highways).

Energy Body

The seven chakras, together with the meridians and acupuncture points located on the meridians form the grid or framework for your energy body. Also, there are energy centers on the palms of the hand and on the bottoms of the feet just below the ball of the foot.

Use the following chart to learn more about the chakras and the effect they have on your body. This chart was abstracted from more detail as presented by Anodea Judith, Ph.D., in her book, *Wheels of Life*. She is a foremost western expert regarding chakras.

7 Major Chakras

Chakra	Sound/Color	Function	Body Parts	Malfunction
Root	Lam Red	Survival, Grounding, Accumulation	Legs, feet, bones, large intestine	Fear Obesity, anorexia, constipation
Sacral	Vam Orange	Desire, Sexuality, Creativity, Physical	Womb, genitals, kidney, bladder, lower back	Guilt Sexual Problems, urinary trouble
Solar Plexus	Ram Yellow	Will, Personal Power	Digestive system, liver, gall bladder	Shame Digestive troubles, chronic fatigue, hypertension
Heart	Yam Green	Love, Self-Acceptance, Peace	Lungs, heart, circulatory system, arms, hands	Grief Asthma, coronary disease, lung disease
Throat	Ham Sky blue	Communication, creativity	Throat, ears, mouth, shoulders, neck	Lies Sore throats, neck and shoulder pain, thyroid troubles
Third Eye	Om Indigo	Intuition, Imagination	Eyes, base of skull, brow	Illusion Vision problems, headaches, nightmares
Crown	No sound Violet/White	Understanding, bliss, connection to spirit	Central nervous system, cerebral cortex	Attachment Depression, alienation, confusion

Energy Centers

The seven major chakras are basically internal discs of swirling energy, acting as the hub or center of multiple meridians of energy. The energy centers on the bottom of the feet and the palms of your hands are external energy centers, enabling your body to receive and release energy.

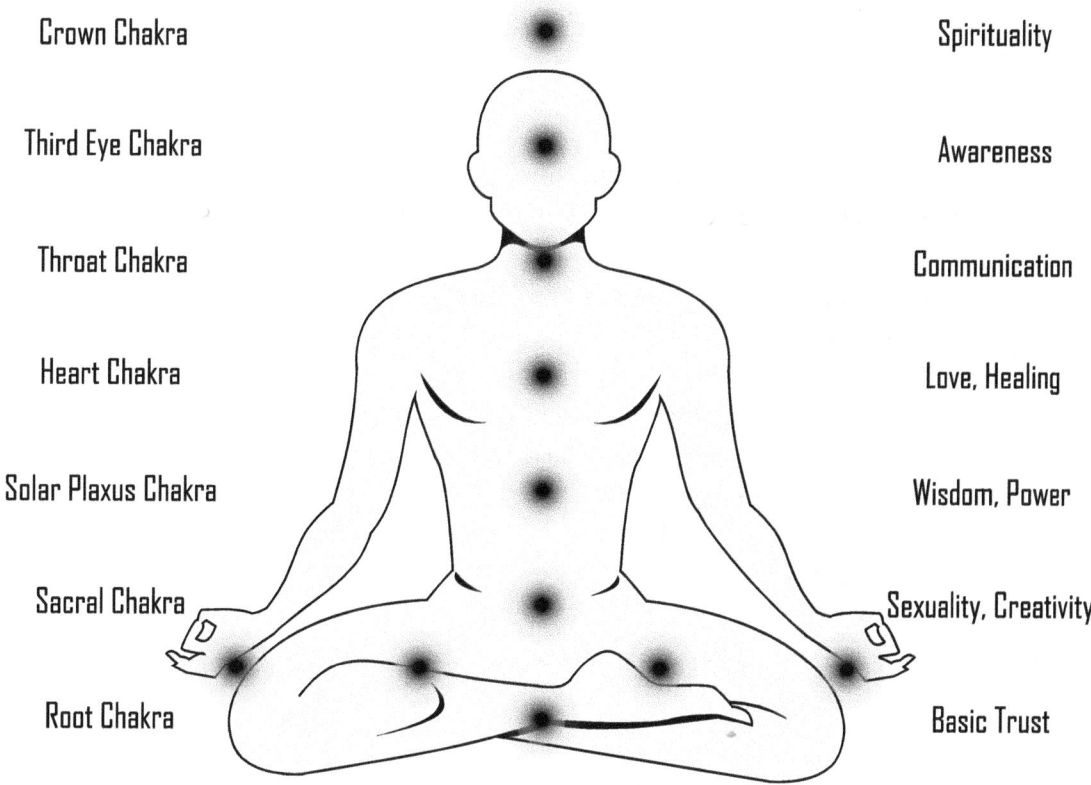

Crown Chakra	Spirituality
Third Eye Chakra	Awareness
Throat Chakra	Communication
Heart Chakra	Love, Healing
Solar Plaxus Chakra	Wisdom, Power
Sacral Chakra	Sexuality, Creativity
Root Chakra	Basic Trust

Summary

Everything you can see, hear, or touch is energy. What appears to be stationery, solid and still is actually energy in motion.

You can think of yourself as a bio-magnet interacting with other bio-magnets within larger fields of energy.

In addition to your physical body, you have an energy body. It consists of:

- Energy centers (seven major chakras basically located along the spine with the crown chakra above the spine on the top of your head and the root chakra slightly below the bottom of your spine}
- Meridians (12-20 major meridians with many minor ones that are basically rivers of energy that carry your life force throughout your body similar to blood vessels carrying blood)
- Acupressure/acupuncture points (hundreds of points located along the meridians; they can be pressed or punctured with a fine needle to relieve blockages)

This was a brief outline of your energy body. The goal is to have your energy body run smoothly without blockages.

If you have a problem understanding your energy body or disagree with my description of these concepts, you can still benefit from the activities. The following chapters describe a number of things you can do regardless of your knowledge or belief systems. Enjoy.

Live well. Do well. Be well.

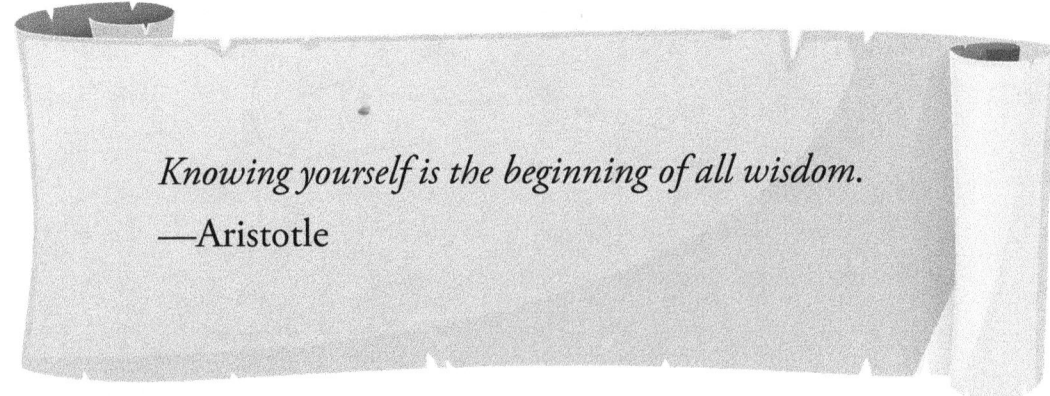

Knowing yourself is the beginning of all wisdom.
—Aristotle

Self

Who Are You? What Do You Want?

These are two important questions you can ask yourself.

1. Who am I?
2. Why am I here? (What do I want? What is my purpose? What do I need?)

To receive answers to these two questions, rely on your inner wisdom. Try the following:

- Stand in a relaxed pose (spine straight, knees slightly bent, buttocks very slightly tucked forward, relaxed neck and shoulders, feet bare or with just socks flat on the ground, arms relaxed and hanging at your sides)
- Close your eyes, and breathe deeply and calmly through your nose
- Take several deep breaths, inhaling and exhaling fully and completely
- Place one hand palm down on your chest over your heart and ask yourself calmly and in a strong voice out loud, "Who am I?" Let the answer come to you (it may not).
- Place your other hand palm down on your lower abdomen (about two inches below your navel) and ask yourself out loud, "Why am I here? What do I want?" Once again, let the answer come to you.

Do not worry if you are not caught up in a vision, exclaiming I am <your answer>. The above is best done after a warmup exercise such as bobbing or tapping or at the end of a full workout and your answers may not come easily. If you do the above each morning after a general warmup you will probably receive many different answers as the days go by. You may think of yourself as a historical figure, define yourself by your relationships to family and friends, see yourself as an energy being, or give yourself a spiritual or religious answer. So, what do you think? Who are you?

During a weekend workshop, a group of us were led through yoga, meditation, and related exercises to answer the question, "What do I really, really want?" Basically, the entire group of participants came to the realization that what they really wanted was to love and be loved. The workshop ended in a group hug. What do you want? Really?

Who are you? What do you want? Why are you here? There are no right or wrong answers, there are only your answers. Ask yourself these questions now, after doing some of the activities in this book, and later, after finishing it. See if you can get into the habit of asking yourself these questions daily. You may want to write down the answers you receive in a log or diary. It is one way of following Socrates' dictum of "Know thyself."

Some would add another question: How do I fulfill my purpose in this life? Mind Valley uses the following three questions when interviewing prospective employees:

1. What do you want to experience?
2. How do you want to grow?
3. How do you want to contribute?

Slomo Shoham tells the story of a Russian mystic who started his daily regimen by swimming nude in an icy, Russian river at 4:00 a.m. every morning. A policeman, new to the region, was making his nightly rounds when he happened upon this long haired, naked man swimming in an icy river in the dark. Astonished, he stopped the mystic, shouting:

- Who are you?
- What are you doing?
- Where are you going?

The wise man regarded him a moment, and then asked him how much he made. The confused policeman told him and the mystic then told the policeman, "I will pay you twice as much if you show up every morning and ask me those same three questions."

Four soul questions discussed by Deepak Chopra in an online seminar:

1. Who am I?
2. What do I want?

3. What am I grateful for?
4. What is my purpose?

So, what do you really want? Who are you? Why are you here?

You Are a Miracle

No matter what your answers are to "Who am I?" you are a miraculous being.

You are a miracle. As a human, you are at the top of the food chain as known on this earth. Your body (especially your brain and heart) are incredibly complex on the one hand and perform straightforward functions on the other. Your brain circuitry has billions of connections, outnumbering the stars in the heavens. Your body has trillions of cells. And this incredibly complex, efficient, effective body/brain complex serves this consciousness called you. Amazing. Simply amazing. Glory in yourself. Be amazed and grateful for the miracle that is you.

Your heart beats 100,000 times a day and your blood travels 3,000 trips each day through 1,000 miles of veins, arteries, and capillaries. Your body is made out of atoms which are at least 99% empty space. You are an almost unbelievable miracle.

Preconceptions

As you try to improve your condition, you may find you have emotional blocks that have been internalized in your body for decades. You may also have limiting beliefs which constrain you. When it comes to being a success or improving your condition in life, your beliefs are more important than your resources.

> *You do not manifest what you want. You manifest what you believe.*

Limiting beliefs and preconceptions may be subtle. You may be embedded in them and not even know it. You may be so attached to your beliefs that it is next to impossible to change them. As a former high school math teacher, I cannot count the number of students who told me, "But I'm not any good at math." In some cases, I spent more time trying to convince students they could succeed at math than I did teaching them math. Most of them still lived their lives, "knowing" they were not good at math.

The real problem with preconceptions and limiting beliefs is that most of them are acquired when you are very young. They are so embedded in the subconscious mind that the conscious mind may not even be aware of them.

Personalities are basically formed by the time a person is five or six years old. More specifically, the brain waves of a person change as he or she grows older. From two to six years old, a child is basically emitting theta waves (deep subconscious for an adult) and imprinting the world on his or her mind/body. By imprinting, the child is accepting the world as sensed and perceived. This is where you get your ideas about who you are, about money and success, relationships, and more. We form our values and as we get older going to higher/faster brain waves, we use our acquired values to accept, reject or otherwise judge what happens to us.

For example, a child may learn that money begets money, the very rich are arrogant and snooty, the love of money is the root of all evil, and so forth. These beliefs can be embedded so deep in the child's subconscious, they are accepted as true and influence the child's entire life. This same child may have a brilliant mind and work very hard but never be able to accumulate wealth and may always be struggling to make ends meet. This could be due to being "programmed" against the rich and riches early in life.

To be really healthy, you may have to change your belief systems. I am still surprised at how healthy I still am and how many years of quality life I may still have. This was not true 10 years ago as I began acquiring the characteristics of the old or what I believed to be the ravages of old age. Letting go of self-limiting beliefs is not easy but it is better than living a limited life. The activities in this book may help you change some of your beliefs, especially those beliefs that are counter-productive to your well-being.

Positive affirmations, especially done in a meditative state, breathing fully and deeply, meditating on a regular basis, and staying or becoming fit using yoga and related activities may all help to open you to a new world of beliefs. These new beliefs may lead you to extraordinary new experiences, including much better health.

Energy Being

Since all matter is ultimately energy, you can be thought of as an energy being. There are two basic illusions that you may experience. These two illusions so permeate Western culture that almost everyone has the following two beliefs which are not really true.

I am Solid

Really? If you remember high school physics, you are composed of atoms which have a nucleus and one or more electrons that revolve around the nucleus. You are composed of trillions of atoms (lots and lots as I do not know what comes after trillions). If one could make a single atom as large as a football field, the nucleus (the solid part) would be about the size of a ping pong ball. That big, large football field would be basically empty. You are a little bit of matter with wide open spaces.

As one writer put it, *"We are 99% empty space."*

I am Separate

Are you sure? Basically, you are an energy field interacting with other energy fields within energy fields. Humans are all part of energy grids interacting with other energy grids that are interacting with other energy grids. In effect, everyone is connected. Some would go so far as to say we are all one and that being separate is an illusion.

Well, what does it all mean? Basically, most people are filled with all kinds of preconceptions, many of which were learned and internalized by the time they were six years old. Many of these preconceptions no longer serve them. Become aware of your preconceptions. Who are you? What do you want? What preconceptions do you need to let go?

Forgiveness

As you question yourself and think about who you are and what you want, and as you examine your preconceptions, some of which may no longer serve you, you may have negative thoughts about yourself, others, or your situation.

I believe each of us should strive to love and accept our self and want to improve our condition and our circumstances. Surprisingly, the first two people I tried to help with the activities in this book told me they could neither love nor accept themselves. This is a mystery to me. Part of the problem is preconceptions.

So many people have low opinions of themselves and do not recognize the miracle that they are. So many people feel unworthy, as though they are here to pass a test and they are failing at it. When I first thought of forgiveness, I thought of aversive parents, bullies, mean teachers, and others, all of whom may have helped imprint you with negative memories and emotions. You may need to be the bigger person and ask for forgiveness from these types of people so you can free yourself from emotional blockages that may be causing you pain and suffering.

You may also need to forgive yourself. If you have feelings of unworthiness, guilt or shame, you may want to forgive yourself for whatever is causing these negative feelings. To acknowledge and accept yourself is basically a prerequisite to becoming well.

The following is a 4-step process to forgiveness first learned through Dahn yoga. It may be a helpful activity to help you forgive yourself and have others forgive you. The four steps to forgiveness:

1. I am sorry.
2. Please forgive me.
3. Thank you.
4. I love you.

When you ask for forgiveness using this method, you are taking responsibility for your negative emotions and releasing them. Increasingly, we know that stress is a major cause of problems with our physical and psychological condition. Much of our stress is due to internalized, negative emotions. This is one way to get rid of them.

You may use these four steps with someone out of your past such as your first-grade teacher, people who are dead, people with whom you had only a brief encounter, and so forth. By going through this process with anyone, including yourself, you are building love and acceptance. This is not a bad thing.

I am Sorry

While in a relaxed state, close your eyes and picture the person whom you are asking for forgiveness. With intent and sincerity say you are sorry for <whatever it is>. If you are working on yourself, you may have several things for which you are sorry and you can do as many as you want in a single session or you can use multiple sessions. If you are asking forgiveness from someone else, there may be a specific incident or situation for which you are sorry. You and the other person may have different ideas of what really needs forgiveness. When you are asking forgiveness from someone else, you may want to conclude with a general statement such as,

> "I am really sorry for any problems, real or imagined, that have come between us and for any pain or negativity I may have caused you."

Please Forgive Me

Taking responsibility for the situation, ask for forgiveness. Whether you are asking for forgiveness from someone or forgiving someone else, you are also forgiving yourself.

True forgiveness is,

> "Giving up the hope that the past could have been any different."

It is letting go of the past you thought you wanted. To find forgiveness is to find freedom.

Another way to look at forgiveness (Dragon Spirit quote from Holly Tse of Foot Reflexology),

> "Forgiveness is giving your heart permission to let go of pain and suffering."

Thank You

Showing gratitude is essential for your well-being. Be grateful for the present and plan for the future with intent and desire. When you thank another person for forgiving you, you are clearing obstacles to your relationship with that person. If you are showing gratitude to yourself, accepting who you are, you are opening yourself to the universe. I like the way Deepak Chopra says it:

> "Gratitude is a state of being in which we feel connected to everything in the universe. It is a fullness of the heart that recognizes the blessings of Nature within and without. Gratitude is love for the goodness of life itself."

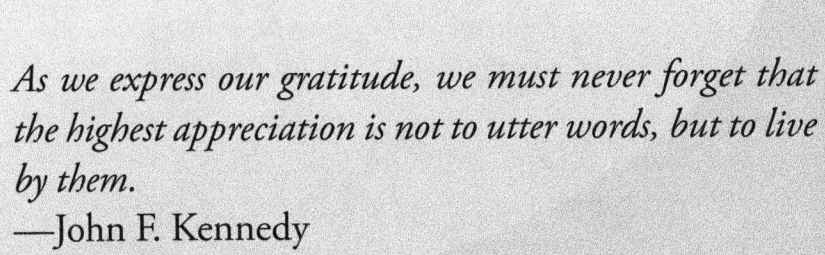

As we express our gratitude, we must never forget that the highest appreciation is not to utter words, but to live by them.
—John F. Kennedy

I Love You

After you have said you are sorry, asked forgiveness, and given thanks for being forgiven, send love to the person you are asking to forgive you.

Love is a basic energy of the universe (some would say it is THE basic energy which is the source or foundation of the universe). When we love someone, it enriches both the lover and the loved.

Try the above four steps with someone you know with whom you may have had a problem or misunderstanding. It feels good to take responsibility for your actions, asking forgiveness, giving thanks and gratitude for receiving that forgiveness, and sending love to the person forgiving you.

Do not forget to forgive yourself. Asking for forgiveness from others and forgiving yourself may lead you to loving and accepting yourself and others. It is a wonderful way to be. Good luck.

Summary

Self-examination and knowing yourself are essential for your personal growth. Who are you? What do you want? Why are you here? Using your inner wisdom, ask yourself these questions often. It is helpful to keep a record of the answers you receive. Over time, you may receive an "ah hah!" experience or two.

Whatever the answers to your questions, you are a miraculous being. You are also an energy being. Wake up to your possibility.

Preconceptions are beliefs about yourself, others, and the world that were usually formed when you were very young. These beliefs may no longer serve you, but are so deep in your subconscious that you may not even know that you have them. Limiting beliefs acquired early and not really true may be causing you grief. As possible, they need to be let go.

One way of asking forgiveness from others and forgiving yourself was included here. By taking responsibility for your perceptions and emotions by saying you are sorry, asking forgiveness, giving thanks, and sending love, you can help free yourself from negative emotions. It is a way to learn how to love and accept others and yourself.

Be forgiving. Know yourself. Be well.

Very little is needed to make a happy life; it is all within yourself, in your way of thinking.
—Marcus Aurelias

Change your thoughts and you change your world.
—Norman Vincent Peale

Thinking

"Thinking is the best way to travel."
—The Moody Blues

Humans are thinking, thinking, thinking.

A human being has 12,000 to 80,000 thoughts a day. It is estimated that about 80% or four out of five thoughts are negative. This constant negative programming is not good for you. It affects your health, attitudes, and perceptions. Even more surprising, it is also estimated that about 95% of our thoughts are repetitive. So not only are most thoughts negative, but they are repeated, sometimes over and over.

When I first saw *The Secret* (iconic video and book that popularized the law of attraction), I came away with the concept: **Thoughts Become Things**.

Your thoughts become things. Think about that for a few minutes. Well, what are you usually thinking? How many of your thoughts are angry, hurtful, or otherwise negative? What are you creating? What behaviors or ideas are you reinforcing?

For me, being positive is sunshine, smiles, and happy thoughts. Positive thinking tends to make people feel good and helps their condition by providing relief from stress and giving them motivation to change. Your attitude and thoughts about yourself affect your health, prosperity, relationships, and all other matters connected to your well-being. Being positive feels so much better than being negative. Studies show that optimistic people live longer than negative people. One study showed this to be 10 years longer. Be happy. Smile. Live long and well.

And yet, so many people tend to be negative in their thoughts, ideas, and actions. Why? These are some reasons why humans are negatively biased.

Humans are negatively wired for survival purposes. When confronted with danger or potential danger, brain centers (the amygdala) control the fight, flight, or freeze response.

When confronted with potential danger, will you fight, run away or freeze like a small animal caught in the headlights of a moving vehicle? This cautious fear of danger may persist throughout your life even when no longer appropriate.

Remembering that your beliefs and preconceptions are basically formed by the time you are six years old, many of your early beliefs no longer serve you. Aversive people and/or a negative environment during your early years can cause you to have negative thoughts throughout your entire lifetime. As you become mindful of your thoughts and actions, a major task is to release yourself from these negative thoughts. Positive affirmations can help.

Is the universe a friendly place? Einstein said that deciding whether or not the universe is a friendly place is a major decision that each of us must make. What do you think? Is your universe a friendly place? In my own life, I have always viewed the universe as friendly or neutral (even when I was ill or injured). I hope you believe the universe is friendly. It seems a better choice than feeling it is not. Believing you are a miracle existing in a friendly universe sounds good to me.

Affirmations

When I began becoming mindful of my thoughts while concentrating on writing about the power of being positive, I was shocked by the negative things I kept saying to myself. Using positive affirmations helped free me from some of these negative thoughts.

An affirmation is a positive statement about yourself or your situation. It can be a goal, belief or desire. It should be positive and not at all negative.

For example, "I am a healthy, happy person filled with love and kindness for all human beings" is a positive affirmation. It is a positive goal or condition. The following is **not** an effective affirmation: "I am neither unwell nor unhappy nor filled with dislike for others." Something like "I will not be so negative with others" is not a good choice for an affirmation as your subconscious may pick up on "will" and "negative" and miss "not" and you may become more negative than when you started.

When creating an affirmation:

- Be positive (say who or what you are or who or what you want to be; do <u>not</u> say what is wrong with you or what you do not want to be)
- Be realistic (an affirmation should be believable and attainable; it can be optimistic; you can also use the words *choose* or *willing* as in "I *choose* to be a loving, kind human" if you're struggling with saying "I *am* a loving, kind human")
- Use repetition to reinforce the affirmation

Although affirmations which are positive, believable (acceptable without backlash from you), and repeated often can help to change your preconceptions and make your life more positive, they are even more effective if they are made at deeper levels of mind. Affirmations done in a meditative state may be more effective than those made during your normal consciousness, when there is so much competition for your attention.

Mirror Work

> The most important mirror principle is:
>
> You must do mirror work to get results. It works in practice, not in theory.

I had done very little mirror work but was drawn to it as a powerful way to make positive affirmations. Louise Hay, a pioneer and leader in both affirmations and mirror-work, credited it for the success, love, and abundance in her life. She used it to overcome self-doubt, low self-esteem and self-defeating behaviors. She emphasizes the use of mirror-work to promote self-love, calling self-love the great miracle cure for healing your life and living a life that truly reflects who you are. When describing herself, she said, "*My originality begins with the thoughts I choose to have.*" Looking forward, she said, "*I choose my thoughts and move into the future.*"

The following excerpts are adapted from some videos led by Robert Holden, Ph.D., and sponsored by Hay House online. To do the following mirror work, he suggests doing each affirmation for a week.

- Sit or stand comfortably
- Maintain eye contact with yourself in a mirror (it can be any size as long as it is large enough for you to maintain eye contact)
- Breathe (normal to deep breathing is good)
- Say the affirmation out loud

> Note: It is effective to repeat the affirmation out loud in a sincere voice with a clear intent. Make several repetitions throughout the day.

Self-Love

Principle: The quality of your relationship with yourself influences all of your other relationships.

Action: Look in the mirror, maintain eye contact, and say aloud, "I love you." Do this for a minute or so (5–10 sincere repetitions with intent) several times a day.

> Note: If you are unable to tell yourself that you love yourself, try "I am willing to love myself" or "I am willing to love and respect myself today" or any positive statement you can make without backlash.

Love

Principle: The mirror does nothing. You do. The world is your mirror; you see things as **you** are. Perception is projection. Change yourself and you experience a new world.

Action: Look in the mirror, maintain eye contact, and say aloud, "Life loves me." Do this for a minute or so (5-10 repetitions with sincerity and intent) several times a day.

> Note: If you are unable to tell yourself that life loves you, try "I am willing to let life love me" or "One way life is loving me today is …"

Intention, Inner Wisdom, Gratitude

Principle: Your life is a mirror; how you experience your life mirrors your beliefs. Every thought you think is creating your future.

Intention: Look in the mirror, maintain eye contact, and say aloud, "I say yes to today." Do this for a minute or so (5-10 repetitions with sincerity and intent) several times a day.

> Note: You can use different affirmations to emphasize your intention. For example, "I am willing to have this be the best day of my life" or "I am willing to let this be the healthiest day of my life" or whatever you want to emphasize.

Wisdom: Look in the mirror, maintain eye contact, say aloud, "What would you have me do today?" Do this for a minute or so (5-10 repetitions with sincerity and intent) several times a day.

> Note: You can ask different questions to trigger your inner wisdom depending on what you want help with in your life. For example, "What would you have me do?" or "Where would you have me go?" or "What would you have me say and to whom?" Per Louise Hay, *"Everything I need to know will be revealed to me when I need to know it."*

Gratitude: Look in the mirror, maintain eye contact, and say aloud, "One thing I am truly grateful for in my life is <what it is>?" Do this for a minute or so (5-10 repetitions with sincerity and intent) several times a day.

> Note: You can be grateful for one thing each day or many things. The important thing is to be grateful for your life. You may also want to keep a journal and write down the things for which you are grateful.

Trust yourself. Loving and accepting yourself, showing gratitude, and relying on your inner wisdom are all good things. The mirror is a safe place to build that trust.

I hope you are inspired to try affirmations, with or without using a mirror. If affirmations resonate with you, check with Hay House, the internet, or your own sources for available books, videos and other materials.

Meditative State

When one meditates, one typically relaxes, let's go of stress, and generates slower, deeper brain waves. While repeating affirmations during an awake state may influence your subconscious mind and help you grow, it is even more effective to make affirmations at a deeper level of mind while meditating. Guided meditations (the leader models and leads you through the affirmations) using affirmations may be a rewarding experience for you.

You can experience making affirmations in a meditative state by saying them as you fall asleep or when you wake up in the morning. Typically, you will be moving into alpha (slower brain waves that characterize the dreaming state of consciousness) as you fall asleep or moving out of alpha as you wake up.

For example, as you are falling asleep, you can affirm, "*Thank you for all of the wonder, joy, and love I experienced today; I am filled with loving kindness and look forward to another day.*" Repeating this in a dreamlike state as you are falling asleep can be a powerful affirmation.

The Meditation section explains the meditative state and slower brain waves in some detail. For now, just know that affirmations done in a relaxed meditative state are more effective than those done in your normal awake state.

Sample Affirmations

As quoted in *The Secret*, Charles Haanel states there is an affirmation that includes everything that a person could want and that the affirmation will bring about harmonious conditions to all things. The affirmation:

I am whole, perfect, strong, powerful, loving, harmonious, and happy.

Basically, the range of possible affirmations depends only on your imagination. Yee Shun-Jian came up with 101 affirmations that he shares on the internet. The following are a few of his affirmations for healing:

- I am strong and healthy
- My energy and vitality are increasing every day
- I am open to the natural flow of wellness now
- Abundant health and wellness are my birthright

- Thank you for my strength, my health and my vitality
- I am feeling stronger and better now
- I love taking good care of myself
- Thank you for the opportunity to balance my mind, body and spirit

Visualization

Closely related to affirmations is visualization. Visualizing what you want to become or what you want to happen is a powerful technique for bringing about desired change. Performing visualization while in a meditative state as you generate deeper, slower brain waves can be really effective.

For example, you may be overweight and want to lose enough weight until you are your ideal weight. You can start with an affirmation such as, "Today, I choose to be my ideal weight." This alone can be effective. During the day you may have a series of negative thoughts such as "I'm so fat" or "I'll never be able to lose weight" and on and on. Every time you start a negative thought about your weight, replace it with the positive affirmation. "Today, I choose…"

You can add a visualization. As you affirm that today you choose to be your ideal weight, you can picture yourself standing on a scale with the scale reading your ideal weight. So now, you can pair the audio affirmation with the visual picture of what you want to accomplish. To be even more effective, you can make the visualization and positive affirmation while in a relaxed, meditative state, which is described in the Meditation section.

Going Deeper

There are several innovations that make positive affirmations more effective.

Mind Movies

These are short clips which combine sound, movement and positive affirmations in an upbeat video. The sound and movement simulate the emotion or desire to change. You can obtain materials to build your own customized videos as well as view a number of completed ones. These are short, upbeat, and a nice way to start the day. They are focused on topics such as Relationships, Money and Abundance, and the like. See Natalie Ledwell and mindmovies.com.

Entrainment

Electronic music designed to bring you to slower, deeper brain waves (alpha/theta) is combined with positive affirmations. Listening requires headphones as this binaural approach uses different frequencies in each ear. Videos may also supplement the process.

Binaural learning is a very powerful tool that works. Be sure you trust the source if you decide to try this.

Guided Meditation

During a typical guided meditation, you are led to a deeper, calmer state of mind. At this deeper level of mind, you may be led through one or more affirmations. In effect, repeating a mantra (Sanskrit sound) is similar to repeating an affirmation.

Affirmations can be increasingly effective as you go deeper into your subconscious mind or otherwise distract the awake, judgmental mind by focusing on the positive.

Contrast

One of the most positive benefits I have received doing positive affirmations is that it made me aware of how negative my ordinary thinking was. I was surprised, even shocked, at how many negative things I said to myself on a regular basis. Replacing negative thoughts (especially those directed at myself) with optimistic, positive affirmations has been a rewarding experience.

A way to free yourself from negative thoughts is to say "Cancel! Cancel!" when you have a negative thought. A recent study reports that optimistic people have healthier hearts and affirmations help people be optimistic. Be happy. Be optimistic. Be healthy. Why not?

Chakra Affirmations

I receive a daily affirmation email from Angela Carter of Bioenergy.com. Each email describes a chakra and gives some action steps to balance it. She provides a daily affirmation to be repeated seven times out loud in a relaxed, quiet environment.

Chakra	Day	Sample Affirmations
Root	Monday	I am supported by those around me. I release all of my doubts and worries. I deserve to be safe at all times.
Sacral	Tuesday	I am peaceful inside. I am grateful for the joy of being me. I am feeling complete peace from within.
Solar Plexus	Wednesday	I am manifesting easily and gracefully. The fire within me burns through all blocks and fears. I am motivated to pursue my true purpose.
Heart	Thursday	I am worthy of the purest love. I forgive myself and others. I am loved because I was born.
Throat	Friday	I honor my opinion. My intent is always clear and noble when I speak. I am an important voice in the world and my voice is heard.
Third Eye	Saturday	I nurture my spirit and am in tune with its need. I am connected to my higher power. I live in alignment with my authentic self.
Crown	Sunday	I remove all limiting thoughts and beliefs. I am open to guidance from the universe. Life will bring me many wonders today.

1. Depending on the day of the week, select one of the above affirmations for that day.
2. In a quiet environment, repeat the affirmation out loud seven times.

Action Steps

The following is a sample action step for the Root Chakra (adapted from Angela Carter).

Look at the trees around you. They've put down solid roots that anchor them to the ground, able to withstand great storms.

Stand with your feet on grass or dirt. If you can, take off your shoes and feel Mother Earth beneath you. Imagine that roots are extending from the bottom of your feet or shoes and attaching deep into the ground, figuratively rooting you to the spot.

You are anchored. Mother Earth will provide for you and yours. These roots also fill you with a sense of security and safety. While you are anchored to the ground in this way, look at the trees and shrubs and flowers that are around you. They too are anchored. Safe and secure.

Just like you.

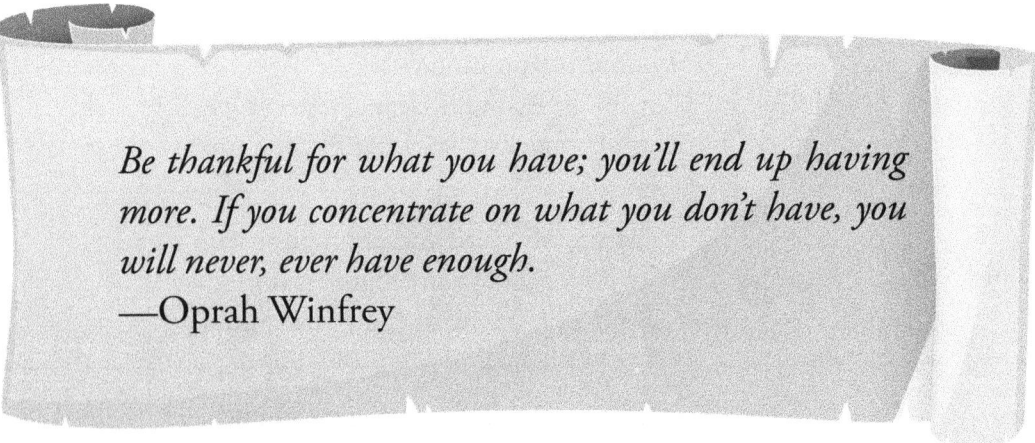

Be thankful for what you have; you'll end up having more. If you concentrate on what you don't have, you will never, ever have enough.
—Oprah Winfrey

Summary

An affirmation is a positive statement about yourself or your situation. It may be what you want to achieve, a truth you want to realize or what you want to become. It is a way to overcome negative chatter in your brain and also a way to let your subconscious mind know what you want.

Done with intention and sincerity, affirmations can help change your attitude, perceptions, beliefs, and actions for the better. If nothing else, it's more fun to think about improving yourself and your situation than going around thinking negative thoughts about what's wrong with you or your situation. A couple of my favorite affirmations:

- Positive thoughts bring me positive benefits and advantages that I desire (Silva)
- Each and every day in each and every way I am getting better, better, and better (Silva)
- I am whole, perfect, strong, powerful, loving, harmonious, and happy (*The Secret*, Haanel)

Your most effective affirmations may be those you create yourself. Just remember: do <u>not</u> include any negativity.

For example, as a writer, "Today, I choose to be creative and productive" may be a useful affirmation. Something like "Today, I will not be stalled by writer's-block" is a not a good choice for an affirmation. If the "not" is missed by your subconscious, you will actually be reinforcing negativity and the idea that you will be stalled by writer's-block. Omit the negative and stay with the positive. It works.

Have fun. Be positive. Be well.

Always remember that you are absolutely unique. Just like everyone else.
—Margaret Mead

Breathing

Breathing well is essential for your well-being and is required to practice yoga and meditation effectively.

Breath is vital to your life. Humans can go weeks without food and days without water but only minutes without breath. Your major physical systems are involuntary (they occur with or without your knowledge or choice such as digestion and maintaining body temperature). Breathing is both involuntary (you breathe automatically when you are asleep or unconscious) and also, under your control. You can hold your breath, deepen it, breathe rapidly or slowly, and otherwise control the way you breathe.

Just as breath is essential for your life, breathing techniques are essential for effective yoga and meditation. Breath is the link or connection between the physical and the spiritual realms. Although only two percent in size, the brain is the biggest user of oxygen in the body (about 20%) and the way you breathe dramatically affects your life.

Breathing and thinking are closely interrelated. Hold your breath for a minute or so. Okay, you can breathe again. Did you stop thinking when you stopped breathing? Many people stop or otherwise have difficulty thinking when not breathing.

Many people in the West breathe too shallowly from the top of their lungs. While exercising, meditating, or just conducting your normal life, aim at abdominal or belly breathing. The abdomen rises on the inhale and contracts on the exhale. If you empty your lungs from the bottom with complete exhales, you will automatically fill your lungs on the inhale. If you are doing only chest breathing you are breathing too shallowly.

Mindfulness Exercise

Try this exercise before continuing.

- Sit quietly with your spine straight. You can be sitting cross-legged on the floor or on a straight-backed chair with your feet flat on the floor.
- Close your eyes and relax
- Simply observe your breathing for a couple of minutes

Do not do anything except watch your breathing. If you have thoughts ripple through your mind, let them come and go. Just observe your breathing. It is your only task. Two minutes. Watch your breathing for two minutes.

Time's up. What did you experience?

Most people report that their breathing slows, deepens, and becomes quiet and regular just by sitting quietly and watching it. Mindfulness (of breath, thoughts, emotions, sensations or actions) is a powerful meditation tool and slow, deep, regular, quiet breathing is required to reach and maintain a meditative state.

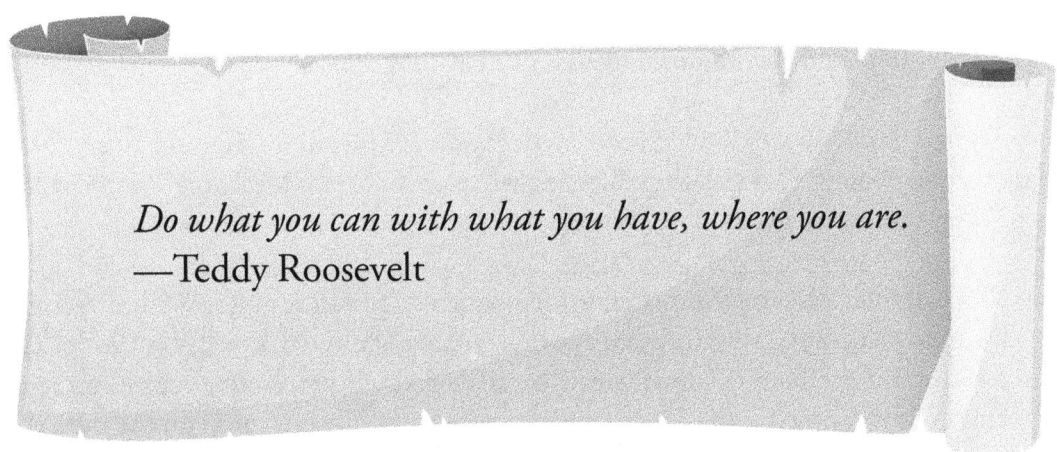

Do what you can with what you have, where you are.
—Teddy Roosevelt

Yoga and Breathing

Having enough oxygen for stretching and holding postures and remembering to breathe completely while exercising is important when practicing yoga.

When doing yoga positions, remember to breathe. When you are intent on learning a new position or listening to an instructor, be sure to keep breathing. You may have a tendency to hold your breath when you are concentrating. Some people do. This is counter-productive. A worthwhile goal is to breathe wholly and fully with each breath.

You may be asked to relax into a stretch. How you breathe can help. Use your imagination to breathe into an area of your body that is resistant to stretching. You can also breathe into an area of the body that is in pain such as a specific joint. Imagine (visualize) breathing energy into the joint and then releasing the pain with the exhale.

You can aid the circulation of energy using your breath. For example, breathe normally, using your imagination to breathe into an energy center, organ or body part. On the exhale, imagine that the excess, stagnant energy no longer needed by you is released through your toes and fingertips.

Some yoga positions require specific breathing techniques to accomplish the exercise. Your breathing is just as important, if not more important, than holding a position or doing a specific yoga movement. Breathe well.

Voluntary

Since breathing is both voluntary (under our control) as well as involuntary (automatic), there are several relatively simple things you can do.

Normal Breathing

- Inhale through your nose
- Breathe from your abdomen (rises on inhale, falls on exhale)
- Focus on the exhale, letting go of unneeded or stagnant energy; you will inhale automatically
- Avoid holding your breath or breathing shallowly; breathe fully with each breath, concentrating on the exhale

Stress Relief

If you are anxious, stressed or feel constriction around your midsection, try some rapid exhales.

- Exhale through your mouth as quickly and as strongly as you can
- Do at least six rapid exhales (it should take seconds, not minutes) before resuming normal breathing
- Walk around and shake any tension out of your system, shaking your arms and hands, your legs and feet

Calming, Energizing Breath

Simply breathing deeply can be both calming and energizing. To do this calming breath, sit or stand comfortably with your spine straight and your hands relaxed at your side. Breathe slowly, deeply, and completely through your nose and then exhale slowly, deeply and completely through your mouth. Just doing this for several breaths will help you to feel calmer and more energetic.

You can take this type of breathing a step further. As you inhale, feel and believe that you are inhaling peace and relaxation. As you exhale, feel that you are letting go of tension and stress. In—relax, out—release, as you continue to breathe deeply. This is an effective way to relax and one way to begin achieving a meditative state.

Using this type of breathing, you can become more aware of the energy you are bringing into your body, its circulation throughout your body, and the release of stagnant, excess, or otherwise unneeded energy.

The following is a simple way to increase your energy and to become aware of the energy in your body. It is adapted from a Qi Gong (energy cultivation) video by Lee Holden. This type of breathing both calms and energizes.

- Sit or stand comfortably with your spine straight and your hands held loosely at your sides
- Inhale slowly and deeply through your nose
- At the top or end of the inhale, pause briefly, imagining your breath changing into energy (Qi or Chi, pronounced "Chee")

- Exhale slowly through your mouth while saying "Chee" softly or in your head
- Continue to breathe in through your nose slowly and deeply, then pause, feeling your breath turn to energy, then exhale through your mouth, softly saying "Chee"
- As you exhale, feel the Qi spread throughout your body
- Do this for a few minutes and then close your eyes and relax completely

How do you feel? Were you able to imagine the energy spreading through your arms and hands? Through your legs and feet? Hopefully, you feel a little calmer and better after doing this type of breathing.

Meditation and Breathing

Breathing during meditation is slow, deep, quiet, and regular. One of the ways to reach the meditative state is to take long, deep breaths in through the nose and out through the mouth. Counting breaths such as taking 10 long, deep breaths before starting a meditation may help you to relax and begin to reach the slower brain waves of meditation.

Many online meditations ask you to take three deep, long breaths before starting the meditation. This, together with soothing music, may help you to reach the meditative state.

Long Deep Breathing

You can do this type of breathing as a stand-alone activity or with yoga or meditation. It is a good way to reap the benefits of abdominal breathing. This activity will help you to learn how to breathe using your abdomen. Inhale and exhale through your nose for this activity.

- Sit comfortably (lying on your back may make this easier)
- Inhale fully and completely
- Relax your neck and shoulders as you inhale slowly, long, and deeply into the abdomen
- Allow your abdomen to fill and expand as your chest rises to fully receive the complete breath

- As you start to exhale, let your chest relax before pulling your navel back towards your spine, expelling all of the air
- Continue this pattern of inhaling and exhaling, placing a palm on your abdomen and feeling your belly expand on the inhale and contract on the exhale

Some Benefits of this type of breathing:

- Cleanses the blood
- Relaxes and calms
- Stimulates brain chemicals (endorphins) that help fight depression
- Regulates the body's pH, which affects the ability to handle stressful situations
- Reduces and prevents the build-up of toxins in the lungs

Healing Breath (4-7-8)

Per Dr. Weil (my source for this type of breathing), it is effective to do a healing breath in the morning upon awakening and in the evening before going to bed. He recommends that you do eight breaths in the morning and eight at night; he emphasizes that you should do only eight healing breaths at a time.

- Sit comfortably with your back straight
- Relax and exhale, clearing your lungs
- Breathe in through your nose for a count of 4
- Hold your breath for a count of 7
- Exhale slowly through your mouth for a count of 8
- Repeat these steps for 8 breaths; do <u>not</u> do more than 8 breaths at a time

Do the healing breath early in the morning upon arising and at night before going to sleep

There are numerous health benefits for this type of breathing. For example, some individuals have had success using the Healing Breath to heal atrial fibrillation. The Healing Breath is part of my morning ritual.

Buddhist Breath/4-Part Breath

For me, this is a simple, quick way to change my awareness. For example, if you are restless, having trouble concentrating, feeling blue or experiencing any condition you want to change, this activity may benefit you. In effect, I use this type of breathing to reset myself, similar to rebooting a computer.

- Sit or stand comfortably with a straight spine
- Breathe in through your nose for a count of 4
- Hold your breath for a count of 4
- Exhale through your nose for a count of 4
- Hold your breath for a count of 4
- Repeat 4 or more times

This is a calming way to breathe. It also helps to change your mind set or consciousness and to still the chatter in your brain as you concentrate on 4-4-4-4.

Breath of Fire

This is a very powerful breathing technique I learned in Kundalini yoga. It can be done as a stand-alone activity or while holding yoga postures.

> **Note**: If you have respiratory problems or related physical conditions, please check with your physician before trying this type of breathing. Do not do this breath if you are pregnant or menstruating.

The focal point of Breath of Fire is at the navel point. It is continuous and powerful. There is no pause between the inhalation and the exhalation. It is a very balanced breath with equal emphasis on the inhale and exhale. The breath is fairly rapid: 2 to 3 breaths per second. In the beginning do <u>not</u> try to go too fast too soon. A slower pace is recommended. Practicing this breath slowly can be more difficult than doing it quickly. Find your balance. Always breathe through the nose, unless directed otherwise.

- When you are starting to learn this breath, focus on the exhale
- As you exhale, push the air out by pulling in the navel point and abdomen toward the spine

- As you inhale, release the inward pull of the navel to allow the breath to automatically return to the lungs
- Place your hand on the abdomen, feeling the inward pull when you exhale, and the relaxation of the abdomen when you inhale
- As you become familiar with this in and out rhythm, increase your speed and inhale/exhale rapidly
- You can do this type of breathing for 1-3 minutes; start with 1 minute and work up to a comfortable length
- If you begin feeling dizzy while doing this type of breathing, stop and take some long deep breaths

Some benefits of the Breath of Fire:

- Strengthens the nervous system to resist stress
- Increases physical endurance and prepares you to act effectively
- Boosts the immune system and may help prevent many diseases
- Releases toxins and deposits from lungs, mucous linings, blood vessels, and other cells
- Reduces addictive impulses for drugs, smoking, and bad foods

During Meditation

In and out, in and out, slow, deep, quiet, regular breaths; in and out through your nose. During meditation, your normal (abdominal) breathing slows and deepens. It becomes quiet and regular.

Focus is the key ingredient to meditating. The following is a simple meditation you can do on your own.

- Sit quietly and comfortably with your spine straight and your eyes closed
- Focus on your breath going in and out of your nose
- Sit quietly and breathe through your nose, observing and feeling your breath go in and out of your nose
- Do not follow your breath into your body, just focus on the breath going in and out of your nose

- If you have thoughts, just let them drift in and out of your consciousness; do not try to repress or suppress your thoughts, just let them come and go and bring your focus back to your breath going in and out of your nose
- If noises in your environment or discomfort in your body cause you to lose concentration or start thinking, just return your attention to the breath coming in and going out of your nose

The above is a simple and effective way to begin meditating. As you strengthen your focus you will be able to meditate more and more easily. Practice the above for several minutes (as long as you remain comfortable and focused while doing it). You may want to get into the practice of doing this short breathing exercise the same time each day. This will help you to get into the practice of doing a daily meditation. Soothing music will also help you to remain calm and relaxed while watching the breath go in and out of your nose.

> Note: This is considered to be one of the most effective ways to meditate. Just watch the breath going in and out of your nose as you sit quietly with a straight spine.

Pranayama & Alternative Nostril Breathing

Most breathing techniques work their roots back to India. For example, the life force, called Ki and chi, is called prana in Hinduism, which means breath. Pranayama is a study of the breath and how to breathe in different ways to reach different states of awareness and consciousness. If you become interested in these other types of breathing techniques, please refer to yoga and meditation books for much more detail.

A widely used technique, alternative nostril breathing is described here. Alternative nostril breathing is a way to experience control and balance in your breathing.

- Sit quietly and comfortably with your spine straight and your eyes closed
- Use the thumb on your right hand to close your right nostril
- Breathe in through the left nostril
- As you complete the inhale, use the index finger on your right hand to close the left nostril while raising the right thumb off of your right nostril
- Exhale through your right nostril

- Inhale through your right nostril
- Close your right nostril with your right thumb while raising your index finger off of your left nostril and exhale through your left nostril
- Inhale through your left nostril and continue as above

We know what we are, but know not what we may be.
—William Shakespeare

People are as happy as they make up their minds to be.
—Abraham Lincoln

Summary

Breathing is essential to your very existence. You can learn to improve your breathing in a class or on your own. As your breath patterns improve, your breathing will enhance your yoga and meditation experience. Normal breathing during yoga and meditation is typically abdominal breathing, although some exercises and movements require special breathing techniques.

When practicing yoga, you can use your creative imagination to breathe into stretches and areas of pain, bringing positive healing energy in through your nose and exhaling pain, stress, and energy that no longer serves you. Simply observing your breath has a tendency to slow, deepen and strengthen it.

There are a number of breathing techniques you can use to achieve a specific purpose. Some techniques such as Healing Breath, Breath of Fire, and Buddhist Breath are included here. Simple quiet, deep, slow, rhythmic breathing is essential for reaching and maintaining a meditative state.

Whether or not you practice yoga or meditation, breathing fully (inhaling deeply and exhaling completely) is good for you. Holding your breath while learning new things or breathing shallowly, is not good for you and can impair physical and psychological function.

Breathe well.

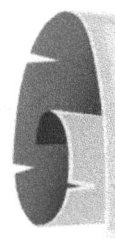

Meditation

This mind-body practice eases stress and boosts mental health. Now, research reveals that it may actually change your brain. One study found that meditating for 2 months increased gray matter in parts of the brain that control emotions and learning. Meditation also strengthens the connection between brain cells. It may also ease inflammation in the brain and protect against Alzheimer's disease.

—Web MD 1/26/22 (certified 8/2/21)

Meditation

There are many systems of meditation and many ways to meditate. It is an inwardly directed personal practice that you can do alone, in a group, or by following a leader during a guided meditation. Meditation has been performed since antiquity in a variety of religious traditions and philosophical systems.

While many people think of meditation as sitting quietly, there are also walking, dancing, and other types of movement meditations used by Sufis and others. Mindfulness (paying attention to the present moment) can be practiced at almost any time while doing almost anything.

Purpose

A basic purpose of meditation is to go to stillness (I think of it as no-mind), to clear your consciousness of thought and clutter. I like to think of meditation as going beyond thought. While this sounds esoteric, the meditation process is simple and beneficial.

Meditation is a way to help you live in the present moment.

Benefits

The benefits of meditation are legion. From helping you to become calm and relaxed, lowering blood pressure, clearing the mind, using more of your brain, solving problems, creating solutions, healing your body, and more, meditation is really beneficial to your well-being.

The following is abstracted from *Buddha's Brain*. Every day there are more studies showing the benefits of meditation.

<u>Regular</u> Meditation has the following benefits:

- Attention
- Compassion
- Empathy
- Increases activation of left frontal regions, lifting mood
- Decreases stress-related cortisol
- Strengthens the immune system
- Increases gray matter in the brain
- Reduces cortical thinning due to aging

Life isn't about finding yourself. Life is about creating yourself.
—George Bernard Shaw

1 Hour a day. Countless benefits.

Give Your Brain a break.

Meditating—even just a few minutes a day—can reduce anxiety and decrease depression.

An hour a day keeps the doctor away.

Meditation decreases blood pressure, lowers cholesterol, and improves immune function.

Make wiser decisions.

Respond with awareness and cultivate a sense of compassion for yourself and others.

Banish stress from your life.

Shed accumulated stress and promote inner calm.

Become the author of your own story.

Go within to rediscover your inner clarity, find your strength, and take back your voice.

Unleash your creative side.

Break out of repetitive thought loops and tap into your brain's deepest potential.

Deepak Chopra – Meditation Class Promo

It helps medical conditions including:

- Heart disease
- Asthma
- Type II diabetes
- PMS
- Chronic pain

It can also relieve the severity of the following:

- Insomnia
- Anxiety
- Phobias
- Eating Disorders

As Mind Valley puts it, the benefits of meditation include:

1. Deep tranquil state.
2. Better health and habits.
3. Free flowing inspiration.
4. Deeper connection with people around you.
5. Mind-blowing sex (Viagra for the soul).
6. Wealth and success (IBM, Mind Valley, and other successful companies are now using meditation).
7. Sense of self-awareness.

Per the American Heart Association, some research suggests that meditation physically changes the brain and could help:

- increase ability to process information
- slow the cognitive effects of aging
- reduce inflammation
- support the immune system

- reduce symptoms of menopause
- control the brain's response to pain
- improve sleep

Classic Pose

Sit in a full lotus (cross-legged with the left foot on top of the right thigh and the right foot on the left thigh) on the floor with your eyes closed or slit slightly open, and your tongue pressed against the ridge on the roof of your mouth behind your teeth with your hands on your knees, palms upward with the tips of your thumbs pressed against the tips of your index fingers is classic. Whew. Well, coming to yoga when I was about 30 with long periods of not practicing it, I have never been able to sit in a full lotus. There are options.

You can sit in a half-lotus (left foot on top of the right thigh or the right foot on the left thigh) or just cross-legged (also called Easy Pose). You can also sit on a pillow (cross-legged or with your legs straight out) or with your back against the wall. Or you can sit on a straight-back chair or even lie on your back on a firm surface. If you sit on a chair, be sure to have both of your feet flat on the floor. This will help to connect you to earth energy. The important point is to keep your spine as straight as possible. At the same time, you must be comfortable to achieve the level of concentration and focus required for a good meditation.

Meditating

When meditating it is good to keep a straight spine (sitting in a chair or on the floor against a wall or even lying flat on your back are all acceptable) to keep your energy centers (chakras) in line. Inhaling should be through the nose; exhaling can be through the nose or mouth depending on the situation.

Given that you keep your back straight (as possible) and inhale through your nose, meditation requires slow, rhythmic breathing and something to focus on in order to occupy your mind.

Breathing (slow, deep, quiet, and regular)

Breathe through the nose. The goal is to aid relaxation and release stress. Breathing should be abdominal (stomach rises and falls as you breathe) or as some say, belly breathing. Your exhale should be at least as long as the inhale and may be up to 1.5 to 2 times as long as the inhale.

If you become frightened or anxious while meditating you may be holding your breath. Fear is a physiological response to not breathing. Relax and encourage yourself to breathe. Take deep breaths, exhaling stagnant, not needed energy. Any fear or anxiety should pass very quickly once you resume breathing.

Focus

Focus is the key to successful meditation. As you become more proficient at meditating, your focus will continue to improve.

Depending on the type of meditation, your focus may be on sound (mantras), sight (mandalas, burning candle, images held in your head such as a buddha or other religious figure), mindfulness (typically of breath while meditating), or on the voice of the person leading you through a guided meditation. As you advance, you may just listen to the silence.

Meditation vs. Contemplation

In Contemplation, you typically use focus and concentration to dwell on or think about a specific event, occurrence, or theme in your life. You can contemplate (think deeply) about almost anything. In Meditation, you focus on something to still or quiet the mind. You quiet yourself as you focus on the object of meditation. Although the processes of meditation and contemplation are similar, in effect, they use opposite channels (thinking and non-thinking).

Monkey Mind

Most people have unending chatter in their heads, always thinking, thinking, thinking. For many of us, this results in talking to yourself as long as you are awake. Other than just distracting you from whatever you are doing, this constant chatter may not help your well-being. Many of us think negative thoughts about ourselves and others, making endless judgments about almost everything.

One goal of meditation is to quiet the monkey mind and ease the endless head chatter. This is not done by repressing or suppressing your thoughts. Instead, simply watch your thoughts as they pass through your consciousness without becoming attached to them. If you are bothered by a monkey mind (and almost everyone is), gently and with purpose, continue to focus on the object of meditation such as your breath or a mantra. Let your thoughts pass through your head as though they were "clouds in the sky on a warm summer day filled with a nice summer breeze."

As you become calmer, more relaxed, and better able to focus on the object of your meditation, you will be able to go deeper into the meditative state. As you go to slower brain waves (alpha/theta) you will be able to focus more strongly. The monkey mind will abate.

On the other hand, it's a rascal. They do not call it a monkey mind for no reason at all. A favorite ruse pulled by my monkey mind is when I'm meditating and I get a thought like "Wow. I'm really doing well. No thoughts have bothered me for quite a while." I'll get caught up in it, and then I'll realize that I'm now thinking and no longer meditating. And so, most people have unending chatter in their heads, always thinking, thinking, thinking... For many of us, this results in talking to yourself as long as you are awake. Other than just distracting you from whatever you are doing, this constant chatter may not help your well-being.

Mantras

A mantra is a specific sound that may be repeated during meditation. It literally means mind tool. Its purpose is to bring you to a certain frequency or state of being. In some ways a mantra is similar to any object of meditation. If thoughts invade your consciousness while repeating a mantra it is best to gently ignore them and to keep your attention on repeating the mantra. A mantra serves a dual purpose: it provides something to focus your attention on and its repetition brings you to a certain frequency or level of awareness.

I have been somewhat wary of mantras (foreign language, what if I'm pronouncing it incorrectly, what does it really mean, and so forth). On the other hand, it is a very beautiful, effective way to meditate. I basically use mantras in guided meditations so I have a model for pronunciation and an interpretation of their meaning. Mantras are effective when just repeated silently in your head. This may be important if you do not want to disturb others in your environment while you are meditating.

Om

Om is the one mantra that is best known in the West and throughout the world. It can be used on its own or in combination with other Sanskrit words to aid you to go beyond thinking, increase your awareness, and experience different states of being.

Om is said to be the primordial sound that was present at the creation of the universe. It is said to be the original sound containing all other sounds, all words, all languages and all mantras. As one author has stated, "Om is the sound the universe makes when it is in harmony with itself."

Om is also spelled "aum" and consists of the three sounds a-u-m. The "a" represents creation, the "u" preservation and the "m" liberation/destruction, which correspond to the Hindu deities Brahma (creator), Vishnu (preserver), and Shiva (destroyer).

It is the universal or prime sound. It may be translated as peace and as yes (affirming what is). To me, it is a safe mantra that has been used for thousands of years and is really helpful. It is pronounced "awwwmmm" or "ohhhmmm" (like the English word "home" without the h sound). You may want to model an experienced meditator when you first start using it. It is a basic, simple, powerful, and effective mantra.

So Hum

This is translated as "I am." You can repeat this mantra silently in your head, saying "So" on your inhale and "Hum" on your exhale. I like it as it's easy to pronounce and a great way to quiet your monkey mind. Try it for a few minutes. To say "So Hum" in conjunction with your breathing requires focus and concentration which helps to quiet your mind.

In a short video, Ich Thant has you visualize energy going from you heart to your third eye as you inhale with the "So" sound and see/feel energy going from your third eye to your heart on the "hum" exhale. You may use this mantra to balance or open your third eye and aid heart-brain coherence.

Sat Chit Ananda

This is one of my favorites. "Sat" ("a" pronounced as "ah") basically means truth or true; "Chit" means intelligence/awareness/consciousness; "Ananda" means bliss. On one of my guided meditations, this mantra was translated as existence, consciousness, bliss. My western mind leapt to, "First we exist, and then we are aware we exist, then we experience bliss." All of the vowels are soft, so "sat" is pronounced "saht (rhymes with what)" and "chit" like the American word, chit. How about "The truth is that I exist and I am experiencing bliss." Whatever its exact meaning, I enjoy the feelings and sensations I have as I repeat this mantra.

Om Shanti Om

In two guided meditations, this was translated as "inner peace" and "I invoke peace." This mantra helps settle your emotions and is soothing for the heart. *Shanti* means "peace," and this mantra has the effect of calming, integrating, and harmonizing the agitation and conflicts in your mind, body, and emotions. The "a" in Shanti is soft like in about; it is <u>not</u> pronounced like "shanty" in English, but closer to "shahntee."

Other

You can use any melodious sound as a mantra. The great wisdom religions of the world are filled with them (Om, shalom, amen, Allah). You can use words with meaning such as peace or love. The Sanskrit sounds, however, have a historical tradition of thousands of years and seem ideal for meditation.

Chanting

Although chanting is similar to using a mantra, it aids total body involvement, may include music and may involve movement. Chanting in a group, especially with people at your experience level or above is a rewarding experience.

I have followed meditations given by Deva and Miten. They are a nice, loving couple and her voice is amazing. Many of the chants they use are quite long and difficult to pronounce. In those cases, I clear my mind, sit quietly and listen with earphones; I do not try to repeat the chant. They use a Tibetan system of repeating a chant 108 times for the 108 energy channels in the body.

I use "Om Shanti Om" as a mantra during meditation and as a chant with Deva and Miten. I do it lying on my back with my hands palm down on my heart or sitting upright with my hands in prayer posture in front of my chest. I attempt to remain true to the Tibetan system by repeating the chant 108 times. You can do this chant aloud or silently in your head. This chant seems to help me clear emotional turbulence and discordant energy throughout my mind and body. I love it.

> *Chanting is a way of getting in touch with yourself. It's an opening of the heart, and letting go of the mind and thoughts. It deepens the channel of grace, and it's a way of being present in the moment.*
> —Krishna Das

Meditative State

Beta	Alpha	Theta	Delta
14-21 cps & higher	7-14 cps	4-7 cps	0-4 cps
Waking state. Five senses. Perception of time and space.	*Light sleep. Meditation. Intuition. No time and space limitation.*	*Deep sleep. Meditation. Creative visualization.*	*Deeper sleep. Unconscious.*

When meditating, you become more relaxed and your brain waves slow.

At any given moment, different parts of your brain are producing brain waves at different frequencies. Your predominant brain waves depend on the state of consciousness you are in. As you meditate and go deeper within yourself, your brain waves become slower and your experiential world changes.

I use the term, meditative state, to refer to the subconscious state consisting of alpha and theta brain waves. It is not important for you to worry about the names or frequency of brain waves; it is important to understand that meditation slows your brain waves, and your awareness changes as you go deeper into your subconscious.

Unconscious State (Delta)

The unconscious state is characterized by very slow brain waves (less than 4 cycles per second) called Delta waves. When you are unconscious, you are in a deep, dreamless sleep with a complete loss of body awareness. I do not know if anyone is able to meditate at this deep level of mind.

Deep Subconscious State (Theta)

The deep subconscious state is characterized by Theta waves (4-7 cycles per second). This level of mind is associated with deep sleep and relaxation. The mind remains active. This is also the level of mind where creative imagery takes place. When you use visualization at this level of mind, the mind does not differentiate between fantasy and reality.

Basically, theta waves require deep meditation and are produced by experienced meditators.

Brain Waves

Your brain waves become slower and regular as you meditate. These are the brain waves when you are awake (beta), in meditation (alpha/theta) and in very deep sleep (delta).

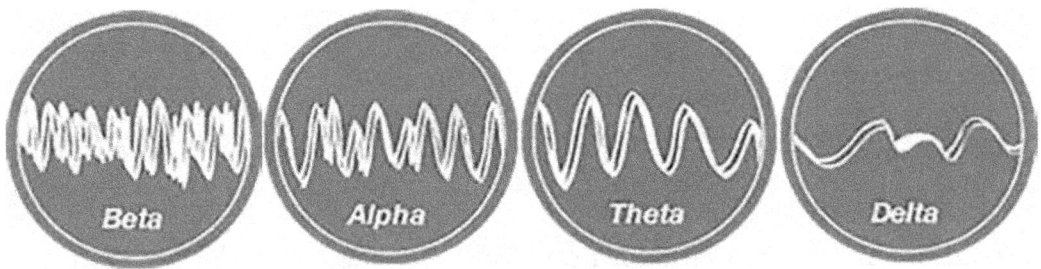

AWAKE - BETA

You are in beta when you are moving, thinking, doing,

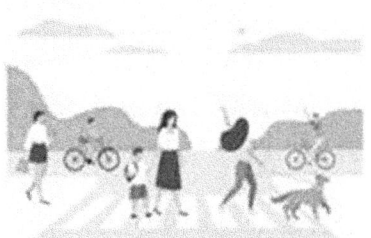

MEDITATIVE STATE—ALPHA/THETA

You are in alpha when dreaming, meditating, lightly sleeping.

You are in theta when you are in deep sleep or deep meditation.

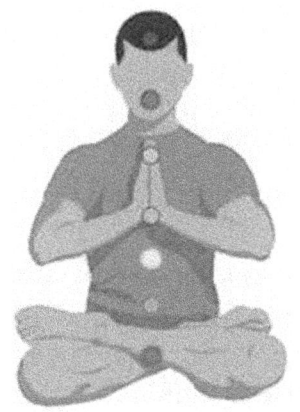

UNCONSCIOUS—DELTA

You are in delta when you are in very deep sleep or unconscious.

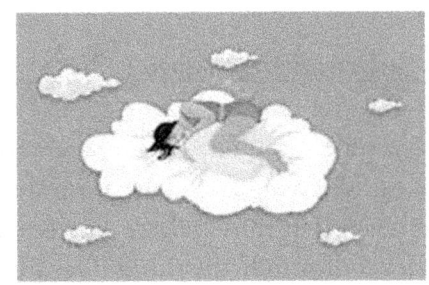

Subconscious State (Alpha)

The alpha state is experienced during light sleep and dreaming. Intuition is enhanced. Alpha waves (7-14 cycles per second) are faster than Theta waves but not as fast as the brain waves experienced during your conscious state. If you watch someone sleeping and their eyelids are fluttering, this means they are dreaming. It is call REM (Rapid Eye Movement) sleep and it is characterized by alpha waves.

For new and intermediate meditators, the goal is to reach the alpha or dreamlike state. You may have experienced alpha waves (7–14 cycles per second) as you are falling asleep or coming out of a deep sleep or if you remember your dreams or wake up during a dream. I used to try and explain the meditative state as being asleep and awake at the same time, although this is not quite true as you remain conscious during meditation.

When you meditate and achieve the alpha state, you are very relaxed and this stress-free relaxation is one of the major benefits of meditation.

Conscious State (Beta)

During your conscious state, you are producing beta (15-30 cycles per second) waves. While you are awake you can use your five senses and experience time and space at the conscious level.

You can also experience your monkey mind, chattering away as long as you are awake.

Observer Mind (Brain waves vary)

In some systems, the observer mind is the fourth level of consciousness (unconscious, subconscious, conscious, observer mind). It is not characterized by brain waves; it represents a way of experiencing or looking at the world.

Observer mind is closely linked to mindfulness. Observer mind is similar to the idea of a "fair witness" that records everything that has happened to you. In Observer mind you simply observe what is happening with equanimity. You neither interfere nor show emotion; you simply watch.

In effect, you stay in the moment by observing or being mindful of your breath, thoughts, emotions, sensations, or actions. Is this important? Humans have the wonderful ability to remember the past and anticipate the future. However, not staying in the present can produce regret, anxiety or other negative emotions and negatively affect your state of being.

What are you doing when you perform routine tasks such as doing the dishes, getting the mail, or being stuck in traffic? Many people think about what has happened to them or what will happen to them. Bring yourself to the moment. Be mindful of what you are doing. Use Observer mind to watch and observe yourself and your environment. Do this with detached acceptance. Do not make judgements. Stay in the present.

Observing what is with acceptance and without judgement will help align you to the universe. Some nice things may start happening for you and to you when you are able to do this.

Mindfulness

The concepts of mindfulness and meditation are basically intertwined. Mindfulness can be traced back to Buddhism. Thich Nhat Hanh points out that Mindfulness is a meditation in and of itself. He emphasizes that Mindfulness is a Way of Being. Jon Kabat-Zinn emphasizes that mindfulness is a way of embracing how you are now. He echoes Hanh, stating that Mindfulness is a formal, rigorous meditation as well as a way of being. Per Wikipedia:

> *Mindfulness is the intentional, accepting and non-judgmental focus of one's attention on the emotions, thoughts and sensations occurring in the present moment.*

One of the easiest and most effective ways to meditate is to be mindful of your breath. Focus on your breath, watching the air go in and out of your nose. As thoughts come up, return your focus to your breathing. Passively notice that your mind has wandered but do it in an accepting, non-judgmental way. You may want to start with short periods of 5–10 minutes or so a day. As you practice regularly, it becomes easier to keep your attention focused on your breathing.

A goal of being mindful is to live in the present. In a Hay House interview, Eric Tolle, a master of NOW, emphasizes that the present moment is all we really have. We can only experience the past as a thought and the future as a projected present. He provides a number of mini-meditations you can do throughout the day.

1. Most of the time.

     You can do conscious breathing, watching the air go in and out of your nose for 15-30 seconds throughout your day. This will help clear some of the clutter out of your mind and give you a sense of being.

2. Bring full attention to something you do often.

     For example, you may be doing errands and getting in and out of your car throughout the day. The next time you get in the car, stop the chatter in your brain. Observe and be mindful of your surroundings, the steering wheel, your body in contact with the seat, and so on. Do this for about 30 seconds.

3. You can do this with any activity that is a means to an end.

     Washing your hands, brushing your teeth, getting dressed, walking up or down stairs are all activities you may do on remote control. The next time you find yourself on remote control, try doing these simple actions with conscious, full awareness.

Some types and aspects of meditation and mindfulness follow.

Middle of the Night—Waking up Restless

You may wake up thinking about the past or future, feeling stressed. This serves no useful purpose. To relieve yourself of this thinking you can focus on your body. Do it from the inside. For example, focus on your hands from the inside. This will take your attention away from your restless thinking.

If the only thing you take away from this book is the understanding and practice of mindfulness, you have done very well indeed. For all of the mantra-driven and guided meditations I have done, being mindful of my breath is still the number one technique I am able to use. Being mindful of my thoughts awakened me to how negative my thinking was and led me to do daily affirmations. Mindfulness is one of the most powerful things you can do.

Goal-Oriented Meditation

Also called dynamic or active meditation, this refers to meditating to achieve a specific purpose or goal. For example, you may want to lose weight, get a promotion, or buy a new car. There are several things you can do in your normal state of mind to help achieve these goals, including thinking, making plans, setting goals, using benchmarks and so forth. You can also use meditation to go to deeper levels of mind in order to achieve specific goals.

While a basic purpose of meditation is to go to "no-mind" while staying in the present in a relaxed state, it has been found that being able to go to the alpha/theta level while being conscious can have profound benefits. For example, you can change habits, visualize success, and help heal yourself more effectively at these deeper levels of mind than while in your normal conscious state.

With intent your conscious mind can tap into your subconscious mind and help you achieve your goals. Positive affirmations are more effective at deeper levels of mind, as are visualizations.

How to do Life Particle Meditation for Manifestation

- Focus on your breath and bring forth an open and sincere heart.
- Create an intention to help yourself and/or others to receive whatever is needed for your (and their) highest well-being.
- Envision a shower of bright, healing Life Particles vibrating in and around you from within the center of your heart.
- Visualize directing Life Particles to yourself, someone else, or situation
- Finalize with your palms placed over your heart in gratitude.

Newsletter@changeyourenergy.com, 5/27/20

Visualization

From a "picture is worth a thousand words" to maps, blueprints, flowcharts, diagrams, and other visual aids such as online presentations, you are probably familiar with the use of visuals to clarify and make a point.

One of the most effective uses of visualization is by athletes to picture and see themselves perform well. Visualization may be used for all sports but can be especially effective for divers, gymnasts, skaters, dancers, and the like. Often quoted, one early study had basketball players practice free throws every day while another group just visualized shooting and making baskets. Both groups did significantly better than the control group which neither practiced nor visualized making free throws. When a Tai Chi master was asked how he could do such complex movements during his Tai Chi routines, he said that first he visualized each movement and once he could visualize all of the steps, he then practiced them physically. He pointed out that the secret to success was the visualization as once a routine was successfully visualized, the rest was just practice.

Visualization is an effective way for the conscious mind to let the subconscious mind know what it wants. Visualizing what you want to happen can be effective at all levels of mind, but it is most effective at the meditative state or alpha/theta level. At the theta level, creative imagery helps shape your reality. At this deep level of mind there is no distinction between images created by your creative imagination or physical reality. In other words, you can use visualization to help move you toward a more positive world and state of being by picturing what and how you want things to be.

Visualization at these deep levels of mind can be made even more effective by including the five senses, color, movement, and emotion. For example, if you want to lose or gain weight, you can visualize yourself standing on a scale reading the weight you want to achieve. To be more effective, you can imagine how your clothing feels, picture yourself in color, watch yourself step on the scale with the scale going from zero to your desired weight and you can be filled with the desire to change your weight. As a final step, you can project yourself into the image in your head and imagine your fitness and joy when you achieve your ideal weight.

To use visualization while in a meditative state, it is probably best to start with a guided meditation. The leader can take you through the process. When you do this type of meditation, your focus is on the voice of the leader. As with all meditation, the goal is for you to focus, stay in the present, and clear your mind of clutter. This will make your visualizations more effective than taking a few minutes a day in between tasks. "Seeing is believing." Good luck.

Entrainment

This refers to the use of electronic music to bring you to a meditative state. While Mozart and similar classical music is relaxing and may help lower and normalize one's pulse due to its melodious beat, entrainment electronic music is designed specifically to bring you to an alpha/theta state. I smile at some of the ads for this type of music: *Zen Buddhist monks take 10-15 years to achieve this deep meditative state while you can do it in five minutes.* They do not mention you will not have the discipline, focus, or training of a Zen Buddhist monk. In a short time, however, this type of electronic music can be both soothing and energizing.

Electronic music (binaural beats) is enjoyable and may help you to relax, reduce stress, and experience slower brain waves while awake. If you are restless, unable to sleep, or anxious, try this type of sound and see if it helps you. Due to the binaural beats, your left and right ears will hear different sounds bringing you to a relaxed subconscious level. It requires you to use earphones to be effective. You can use this type of sound to energize and focus yourself, helping you achieve what you want.

> Note: Using binaural beats is a very powerful technique that is gaining popularity. Audio tapes are designed to lead you to specific outcomes. Please be sure to use trusted sources for this type of activity as it is very powerful.

Osho Says

The following is a glimpse at a deeper, more profound view of meditation.

Osho is a mystic who passed away in 1990. He presented meditation not only as a practice but as a state of awareness to be maintained in every moment. He viewed meditation as a total awareness awakening the individual from the sleep of mechanical responses conditioned by beliefs and expectations. The following are some of his daily quotes from a 21-day meditation for busy people sponsored by Mentor.

> *"Meditation is the breath of your soul. Just as breathing is the life of the body, meditation is the life of the soul."*

> *"When mind knows, we call it knowledge. When heart knows, we call it love. And when being knows, we call it meditation."*

"This is the way of meditation: encountering the present in all its tremendous beauty."

"When consciousness is empty of all contents, that's what we call no-mind or meditation."

"Silence is the space in which one awakens, and the noisy mind is the space in which one remains asleep."

Guided Meditation

Enjoying online meditations, I immediately tried to get everyone I knew to try them. My excitement and attempted sharing were met with a loud thud. Perhaps Osho was right about why people did not get into meditation.

"If you feel much resistance against meditation, it simply shows that deep down you are alert that something is going to happen which will change your whole life."

In my frustration, I was reminded of advice I received in a workshop,

"Do what you think and feel is right; do not be attached to the results as they may not live up to your expectations. Just continue to do what is right."

Deepak Chopra, together with Oprah Winfrey (and other guest presenters), has done several 21-day meditations online. The guest introduces the topic, providing personal insight and inspiration, and Deepak goes deeper, discussing the centering thought for the day and introduces and models the mantra to be used. The rest of the time is spent meditating on the mantra.

There are many other online meditations which are available. Many are really good and very worthwhile. They are free, but do require a time commitment. To start your meditation practice, I would suggest practicing mindfulness, especially of your breath, then doing a short (5-10 minutes) meditation at about the same time each day. You can then expand your meditation practice to guided meditations, either online or with a local yoga or meditation group.

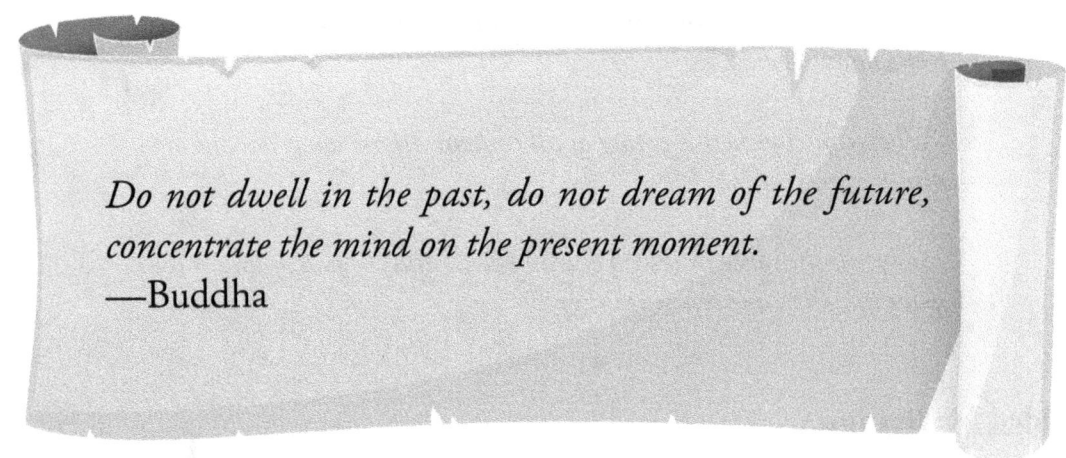

Do not dwell in the past, do not dream of the future, concentrate the mind on the present moment.
—Buddha

Chakra Healing

The seven major chakras (crown, third eye, throat, heart, solar plexus, sacral, and root) discussed in the Energy section are the hubs or centers of energy in which the major meridians or paths of energy flow. To achieve optimal health and well-being, the seven chakras (pronounced shock-rah, sort of) should be open and balanced. I would suggest you use a guided meditation by someone you trust to help you keep your chakras open and functioning well.

This is a relatively simple meditation that you can use to start the process of having healthy, open energy centers. As desired, play some soft, melodious music (this can also be ocean waves, soft rain, or nature sounds). In this meditation, you are just going to scan your body and acknowledge how it feels. You do not have to actively try to change anything. Awareness brings change. This meditation helps you become aware of your body.

- Achieve a meditative state by doing <u>one or more</u> of the following (whatever works for you)
    - Take 10 deep breaths, counting them as you slowly breathe in and out, OR
    - Take 3 deep breaths, while inhaling slowly and deeply through your nose, imagine your mind and body being filled with peace and relaxation; while exhaling slowly and deeply through your mouth, imagine letting go of any stress or tension in your mind or body, OR
    - Count backwards from 100, 50, or 25 to 1, assuring yourself that when you reach the number one you will be in a meditative state, OR

- - Sit quietly, watching your breath go in and out of your nose, OR
  - Use a mantra such as OM
- As you relax into a meditative state, sit quietly with your spine straight, scan your body and its chakras (energy centers)
- Scan the root chakra, located on your pericardium between your womb or genitals and rectum, a few inches below the end of your tailbone, and the body parts it governs. Scan your legs, feet, bones, and large intestine. How do they feel?
- Scan the sacral chakra, located about two inches below and in from your belly button, and the body parts it governs. Scan your womb or genitals, kidneys, bladder, and low back. How do they feel?
- Scan the power chakra, located a couple of inches above your navel and below your sternum, and the body parts it governs. Scan your digestive system, liver, and gall bladder. How do they feel?
- Scan the heart chakra, located in the center of your heart, and the body parts it governs. Scan your lungs, heart, circulatory system, arms, and hands. How do they feel?
- Scan the throat chakra, located in the center of your throat, and the body parts it governs. Scan your throat, ears, mouth, shoulders, and neck. How do they feel?
- Scan the third eye, located in the center of your forehead, slightly above your eyebrows, and the body parts it governs. Scan your eyes, base of skull, and brow. How do they feel?
- Scan the crown chakra, located at the top of your head, and the body parts it governs. Scan your central nervous system and cerebral cortex. How do they feel?

When you finish scanning your energy centers and the parts of the body they govern, you can sit quietly and be aware of the air going in and out of your nose. How do you feel? If your attention is drawn to a specific part of your body, this may indicate you need to do something for this physical area.

You can also meditate on individual energy centers, using their sound (such as lam, pronounced like the "a" in father, close to lahm for the root chakra) or their color. Refer to the chart in the Energy section for a complete listing of the sounds and colors associated with the chakras.

Dahn yoga uses different colors (red, orange, yellow, green versus red, reddish-orange, orange, yellow) for the lower four chakras (the upper three of sky blue, indigo, and white/

violet are the same) than Hatha or Kundalini yoga. Many people do not see colors or they see radically different colors than other people. Everyone has their own filters. If it is helpful to you, you can use colors to help you meditate on a specific energy center. Otherwise, it is not necessary to picture a specific color.

By meditating on a chakra, you bring energy to it which may have curative powers and help your well-being. If you are having serious problems with fear, shame, grief or other negative emotions associated with malfunctioning energy centers, you may want to seek some professional help and guidance.

Energy Meditation

When leading Energy Meditation Circles, this was the beginning meditation I used. It is a good way to become sensitive to the energy coursing through you and can lead to a very powerful meditation experience.

- Sit quietly and achieve a relaxed, meditative state by taking several deep breaths, or whatever works for you (do not worry if you do not automatically go into a deep, alpha/theta state; just take some deep breaths and then sit quietly and watch the breath go in and out of your nose)
- Activate your hands by rubbing them vigorously until they are warm
- Hold your hands in front of your chest about 2-4 inches apart in a modified prayer posture (palms and fingers facing each other)
- Be aware of your hands (do you feel a tingling or heat in your hands?) and the space between them
- Very slowly and gently let your hands move apart as you inhale and move closer together without touching each other as you exhale
- Imagine that you are holding an energy ball that becomes larger as you inhale and smaller as you exhale
- Sitting in a quiet, still state with your eyes closed, you can begin playing with your energy ball. Is it the size of a tennis ball, a basketball, or is it larger or smaller?

From this initial state of holding an energy ball in front of your chest, there are many things you can do on your own, although you may want to find and use a teacher.

Simply visualizing an energy ball in between your hands in front of your chest that expands and contracts with your breath is a nice meditation in itself. Try doing it for 5-10 minutes and see how you feel. Over time you should become increasingly sensitive to the energy in between your hands and this meditation becomes calming and relaxing.

Imagine/visualize/feel the energy ball getting larger and larger until it encompasses your whole body; in effect, see yourself in a large bubble of healing energy that enhances your well-being. This ball of energy can then grow to encompass the whole room or area where you are, the community, the country, the world, and beyond. It can be a nice way to express your love for yourself and others.

> Note: If you are doing this type of meditation in a group (typically sitting on the floor in a circle), you can do a group bubble, with all participants creating it.

1. Bring the energy ball into your body (typically through one of your energy centers such as the sacral chakra). In your mind's eye, roll the energy ball up the back of your spine to the top of your head and then down the front of your spine. Repeat this three times. This is a great way to aid circulation and gain some control over the energy in your body.
2. Bring the energy of the energy ball into your body. For example, in group energy meditations, participants hold the energy ball a few inches above the top of their head, imagining a steady stream of energy descending from the energy ball through the crown chakra and filling their entire body. Once the energy ball is stable, participants can let down their hands and continue to imagine this pure, clean, healing energy filling their entire body, starting from the head and going to the toes. You can also imagine that each and every cell of your body is filled with this wonderful, pure, healing energy and that you are becoming totally rejuvenated.

There are many types of energy meditations with similar but different processes and outcomes. I recommend that you use or find a teacher/leader if energy meditations feel right for you.

How to meditate? There is no need to ask how to meditate, just ask how to remain unoccupied. Meditation happens spontaneously.
—Osho

Summary

Meditation is a way to be in the present, clearing the mind of chatter and clutter. It has traditions dating back thousands of years and has been used in a variety of cultures. Its benefits are legion, ranging from experiencing a deeper, more relaxed state to achieving specific goals.

To meditate, deepen your breathing (slow, regular, and rhythmic) and focus (for example, on a mantra/sound, your breath, or instructions from a guide). Be aware of but do not attend to thoughts, emotions, or bodily sensations which may arise. Continue to breathe slowly and deeply while continuing to focus on the object of your meditation. Remember to be playful and have fun.

The meditative state (slower brain waves typical of the alpha/theta subconscious states) is a wonderful way to relax. You can also amplify the effects of visualization, affirmations and goal-oriented focus when you are in a meditative state.

Sitting quietly, relaxed, with a straight spine while watching the breath go in and out of your nose or while chanting a mantra sounds good to me. Enjoy doing this. Do not worry about the chatter in your brain or anything else that prevents you from meditating. Try it a little each day. It gets better and more rewarding as you learn to relax and focus.

Relax. Enjoy. Prosper.

Hands

Most of our nerve endings are located in the face, hands (palms), and feet (soles). The hands may be used to experience the energy of your body, help distribute energy to different areas of your body, and help heal yourself and others. Hand gestures are used in both yoga and meditation, called mudras in Hinduism and Buddhism.

Warm-up Exercises

To warm up your hands or activate the energy in them, you can do any of several things:

- Shake them vigorously
    - In a standing or comfortable sitting position, shake both hands vigorously
    - You can shake your hands while holding them waist high, at chest level, over your head, or wherever it feels right
- Rubbing
    - Rub the palms of your hands together vigorously
    - Rub them as fast as you can, feeling the heat
    - Do this for a couple minutes or until they are very warm
- Clapping
    - Do this strongly but not to the point of discomfort
    - Clap your hands together 10-20 times, be sure to include the palms and all of your fingers
- Screwing in a light bulb
    - Hold your hands slightly over your head and pretend that you are screwing in two light bulbs
    - Do this vigorously for a short period of time; you may feel your fingers become thick like sausages and filled with energy
- Knuckles
    - Hold your hands in a loose fist
    - Rub the fingernails and first knuckle of each hand together for a few minutes

After activating your hands using one or more of the above methods, stand comfortably with a straight spine, your feet shoulder width apart and your knees slightly bent. Let your hands hang loosely at your sides. Close your eyes, breathe through your nose and feel your hands. If you have activated the energy in them, you may feel tingling, warmth, or other sensations.

This is one way to begin to be aware of the life force energy (Ki, Chi, or Qi) coursing through you. It is also a good start to giving yourself or someone else a massage. You can also use hand activation as the start of an energy meditation.

Palming

Once your hands are warm and activated, try palming. Lie down flat on your back (use a pillow as desired), close your eyes and cover them with the palms of your hands. You can also do this while sitting or standing. Make sure you are in a comfortable position and do this for at least a few minutes. You can do this as often as you like for as long as it is comfortable. While you are palming, you can also do eye exercises with your eyes open or closed while completely covered by your palms (no light). When you are done palming, your eyes will be more relaxed and things will be a little brighter.

- Activate (rub) your hands together until they are warm
- In a comfortable position, close your eyes, and cover them with the palms of your hands
- Rest comfortably, feeling the energy in your hands interact with your closed eyes
- Optionally, do eye exercises while your eyes are completely closed and covered
    - Look up, look down, look to the right, look to the left
    - Rotate your eyes clockwise
    - Rotate your eyes counter-clockwise

When palming, you can take the opportunity to watch the breath go in and out of your nose. It's always calming to be in a meditative state. Palming can help you relax your eyes and relieve any tension you may have around them. It feels good and it is enjoyable.

3-Finger Technique

Learned initially from the Silva Method, this is a simple way to help you remember something such as, "Where did I leave my keys?"

- Sit or stand in a comfortable position, focused on what you are trying to remember or do
- Press the pads of your thumb, index finger, and middle finger together (I tend to use my right hand but you can use either or both hands)
- Say aloud or silently to yourself what you are looking for or attempting to remember

You can also use the 3-finger technique to focus your attention. For example, you may find this technique helpful to locate a parking place, find a product at a grocery store, or to make minor decisions. The 3-finger technique helps you to focus, and can be helpful when you have forgotten, misplaced, or cannot find something.

Acupressure Points

An acupressure point is like a bus stop along the highways of energy called meridians in your body. These points may be used for acupressure (pressing or putting pressure on them activates them) or acupuncture (a skilled professional uses small needles to open them).

A blocked acupressure point acts like a traffic jam. Putting attention and pressure on blockages brings your energy there and helps open and release the flow of energy along the meridian.

Hand Crease

There is an acupressure point in the crease of the hand in front of where the thumb and forefinger meet on the top of your hand. When you press down at this point, you may feel some tenderness or pain. Putting pressure on this point helps relieve headaches. Some people report feeling the energy of a tension headache drain out of their head into the hand as they put pressure on this point. It appears that this point works well for relieving tension headaches and hangovers.

If you have trouble finding this point or activating it, try this.

- Take either hand and fold the thumb into the palm
- Use the other hand to deliver a karate chop (small finger side of the striking hand) to the crease of the hand you are working on
- Do this gently but firmly several times until you feel that this pressure point is open
- As desired, switch hands and repeat the above

There are hundreds of acupressure points, each of which affects our well-being. If you become interested in acupressure or acupuncture, contact a certified practitioner.

Pledge of Allegiance

If you place your right hand, palm down on the left side of your chest angled to the left as though you were pledging allegiance, and press down with your fingertips you may be able to locate an area of nerve endings which will be sensitive to your touch. This area is between your collar bone and your nipple, about ⅔ of the way toward the collar bone. Keep probing, when you find it, you will know it.

- With your hand on your chest, this is a good time to activate these nerve endings while doing positive affirmations:
- Place your right hand, palm down on the left side of your chest as though you were saying the pledge of allegiance
- Probe with your fingertips until you locate a sensitive area of nerve endings (about ⅔ of the way between your nipple and collarbone)
- Maintain pressure on this area with your fingertips while doing positive affirmations such as:
    - I deeply love and accept myself
    - I am willing to love and be loved
    - I choose to be healthy, happy, and filled with loving kindness for all

Activating these nerve endings will increase the positive effects of your affirmations.

Mudras

A mudra is a hand gesture that you may use in yoga and meditation. Some of them are quite simple and beneficial. After my accident, I could not walk for three months and used hand gestures while trapped on the couch.

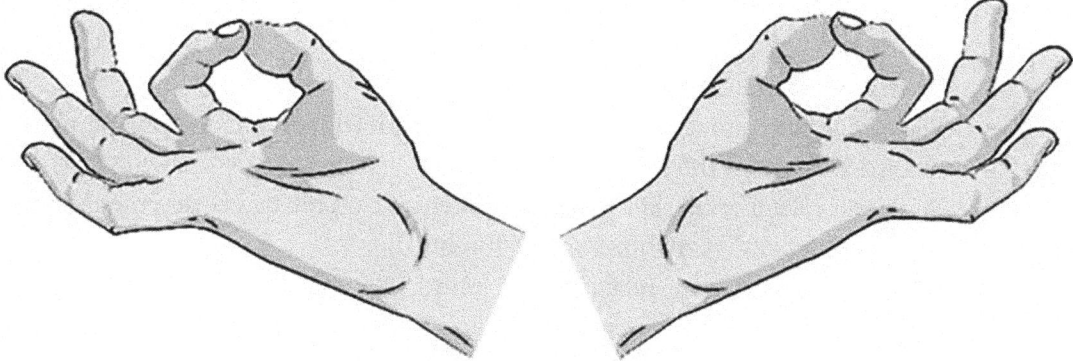

- This hand gesture is used in the classic meditation pose (sitting on the ground in a full lotus, half-lotus or cross-legged).
- Join the tips of your thumb and forefinger on each of your hands, forming a circle while extending the rest of your fingers
- Place your hands palms-up on each of your knees or thighs while sitting in a meditative pose (cross-legged on the floor or sitting in a straight-back chair)
- This mudra activates your diaphragm, making for deep "stomach-breathing" as the diaphragm pushes out the internal organs when it descends towards the pelvis on inhalation. While in this classic pose, you can practice slow rhythmic breathing in a 5-2-4-2 rhythm (exhale for a count of 5, hold for 2, inhale for 4, hold for 2, repeat). This enables prana (life force) to flow in your pelvis and in your legs.

You can use this hand gesture in basically any meditation with any type of breathing.

Prayer Pose

The universal symbol of prayer (palms together in front of your chest with your fingers pointing upward) has been used worldwide by saints and sages of many cultures and spiritual traditions. It may be referred to as the Mudra for Divine Worship. Connecting the palms and fingertips symbolizes unity and oneness and magnifies your healing.

- Sit in a comfortable position
- Place your palms together in front of your chest (fingers facing upward, elbows relaxed and out to the side)
- With eyes closed or slit slightly open, concentrate on the third eye (point between the eyebrows and ¼ inch up on the forehead)
- Breathe long and deep, relaxing your mind
- Continue for at least three minutes

You can use a mantra such as Om to further focus your consciousness while doing this hand gesture. The goal is to become totally at peace with yourself and the universe.

Hakini Mudra Hand Position

Use this mudra to help create a sense of calmness which opens your mind to clearer thinking and helps you put things in perspective.

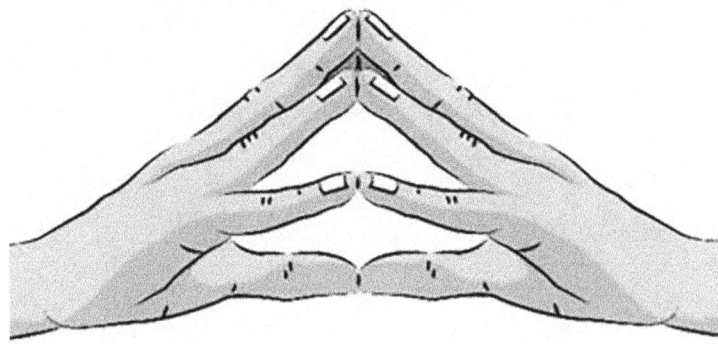

Hakini Mudra balances the left and right hemispheres of the brain. The left hemisphere of the mind does logical thinking and the right half is about creativity and memory. This mudra opens access to the right hemisphere where memory is stored. It helps boost thinking while improving concentration and memory.

Hakini Mudra

Hakini Mudra also builds up the energy in the lungs and improves and deepens respiration. It activates the 6th Chakra or Third Eye which is the point of your intuition.

- Hold your hands open facing each other, with the fingers spread apart
- Place all of your fingertips together with the fingertips and tips of the thumbs touching
- Do not touch your palms together
- Focus on whatever you are trying to remember or want to concentrate on such as your work, what you are reading, or taking an exam
- Practice long, deep breathing while using this hand gesture
- Continue to practice this mudra for a few minutes or until you reach your desired effect

You can practice this Mudra while sitting, standing, lying down, or walking. It can be quite useful for recall, such as remembering a person's name, where you left something, a restaurant where you dined, or a movie you saw.

For recall, you can add the following to the steps above:

- Inhale, placing the tip of your tongue on the roof of your mouth behind your teeth
- Exhale, while releasing the tongue
- Practice this for several breaths
- To finish take a couple of long deep breaths
- The memory may come right away or take some time

This mudra can also be beneficial when you are traveling and feeling a bit far away from home or have a longing or a pull to be home but wish to continue on your journey. As an option, you can do the following for more grounding:

- Hold the mudra in front of your heart center in the middle of your chest
- Your eyes may be open or closed: if closed keep your eyes focused on the Brow Point in between the eyebrows about a ¼ inch up
- Practice long deep breathing
- Continue this for 3–5 minutes or as long as needed

Joint Mudra

The Joint Mudra balances energy in your joints and helps with stiffness, soreness, and pain. It can help restore, balance, and heal the area in and around the joints. If you have a job where you sit for long periods of time and/or have become less active this mudra would also be of benefit to you. As time goes on, this process can help facilitate movement.

- On the right hand, press the pads of the thumb and ring finger together
- On the left hand, press the pads of the thumb and middle finger together
    - Right Ring—RR
    - Left Middle—LM
- Keep your other fingers relaxed and straight out
- You can hold this mudra while sitting in a comfortable position, going for a walk, watching television, or other times when your hands are free. No Driving. Please.
- Breathe normally for the entire time, or as an option, you can use a long deep breath imagining yourself breathing into the area you would like to heal for the first few minutes, then resume normal breathing
- Practice this mudra for 15 minutes, 2–4 times a day or as needed

This mudra is subtle and the healing may take months so stick with it and you can have a favorable outcome with good results. I found out about this mudra from my Kundalini collaborator. I began combining it with my evening and morning meditation and have practiced it religiously for months. It is subtle but I love it. It helps relieve my morning stiffness. My experience with the Joint Mudra moved me to include hand gestures in this book.

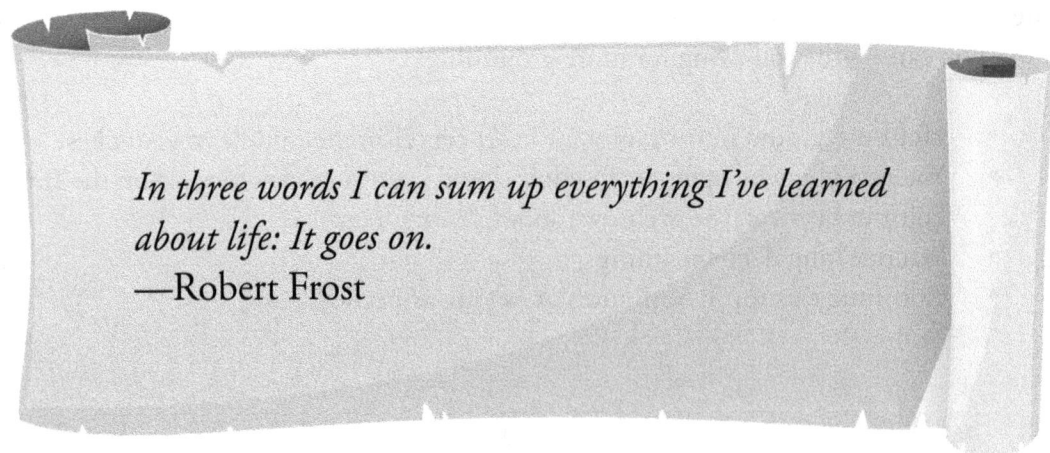

In three words I can sum up everything I've learned about life: It goes on.
—Robert Frost

Mudras for Calm and Patience

You can use both of these mudras for helping you to settle down and put things in perspective.

Gyan Mudra (passive)

- Join the tip of the thumb with the tip of the index finger using consistent, firm pressure
- Press on the fleshy part of the finger and not the fingernail
- Breathe normally or long and deep while using this hand gesture Use this for calmness, receptivity and to stimulate knowledge and wisdom.

Shuni Mudra

- Join the tip of the thumb with the tip of the middle finger using consistent, firm pressure
- Press on the fleshy part of the finger and not the fingernail
- Breathe normally or long and deep while using this hand gesture.

Use this for patience, discernment, and the ability to commit.

Restless Night

If you wake up during the night and find yourself worried, anxious, or fearful try these hand positions. These are from Jin Shin Jytsu, an ancient art of harmonizing the life energy in the body. Relatively obscure, this philosophy was revived in Japan in the early 1900s and brought to America in the 1950s. These hand gestures are quickies to help you settle down a bit and can be used whenever you become worried or fearful.

Thumb—Worry

- Wrap the fingers and thumb of your right hand around the thumb of your left hand
- The fingers of your left hand can be out and relaxed or gently resting on your right hand
- Hold this position and breathe; you may breathe normally or practice long deep breathing
- After a period of time, switch hands holding the right thumb with your left hand
- You can also switch back and forth. Give yourself plenty of time on each side

Do this until you are feeling calmer and more connected.

Index Finger—Fear

- Wrap your fingers and thumb of your right hand around the index finger of your left hand
- The fingers of your left hand can be out and relaxed or gently resting on your right hand
- Hold this position and breathe. You can breathe normally or practice long deep breathing
- Switch hands holding the right index finger with your left hand
- You can also switch back and forth. Give yourself plenty of time on each side

As with the Worry mudra, do this until you are feeling calmer and more connected.

Summary

The palms of your hands, together with your face and the soles of your feet are filled with nerve endings.

Your hands can be activated (filled with energy) by rubbing, shaking, or clapping them together. As explained further in the following Yoga-Related Activities section, they can then be used to distribute energy to different areas of the body through tapping and massage.

Palming is a way to relax and energize your eyes.

Hand gestures (called Mudras) are used in both yoga and meditation with some examples included here. You can use Hand gestures to center and relax yourself, as well as help bring about desired outcomes such as better joint circulation.

For the most part, these are simple exercises that can be done while sitting or confined to a bed. Relax. See which ones are helpful and do them as often as you like.

These simple hand gestures can help your well-being. Try them. Use the ones which feel good.

There is only one corner of the universe you can be certain of improving, and that's your own self.
—Aldous Huxley

Yoga-Related Activities

I think of the activities in this section as yoga-related. I have learned or participated in all of them in yoga classes except for EFT (Emotional Freedom Technique) which uses meridian tapping. Some of them are warm-up techniques. All of them will help you relieve stress and are good for you physically. They are mostly straightforward and should be helpful to help relieve and lessen emotional or physical pain.

Simple Is, Simple Does

These are some relatively simple exercises that may bring you immediate benefits.

Tapping

Tapping your body aids circulation, helps reduce stress and tension, and helps remove or minimize energy blockages. It is simple and can be extremely helpful.

You can tap your body by using your fingertips, cupped hands, or loosely held fists.

Using your fingertips to tap is especially effective when you tap on parts of your head or along your major meridians. You may use your two fingers (index and middle), all four fingers, one hand or both hands.

Tapping your head with your fingertips, start by tapping the crown of your head (location of your crown chakra or highest energy center), then the sides of your head, the back of your head (giving your brain stem a nice workout), around your ears, then your forehead and face. Tapping around your eyes (the bone ridges just above your eyes, to the sides of your eyes, and just below your eyes) is a good way to ease tension and may help you relieve tension headaches. If tapping your temples is painful you may have liver or anger issues.

The tapping, itself, is rhythmic and should be at a pressure that is comfortable for you. You can do head tapping on your own. Meridian tapping should probably start with a teacher. A teacher or energy healer can tap your meridians, show you where and how to tap, and provide feedback when you try tapping. EFT (Emotional Freedom Technique) is a form of meridian tapping that is becoming increasingly popular. It is described later in this chapter.

When using cupped hands to tap, you can tap anywhere on the body.

- Stand in a comfortable position (feet shoulder width apart and facing forward like an 11, knees slightly bent, shoulders and torso relaxed, hands loose and relaxed at your sides)
- Cup your hands and rhythmically slap the palms of both hands on your lower belly at the same time, one hand on each side of your lower abdomen
- Let your knees bounce up and down as you tap your lower belly using both hands at the same time
- Continue this type of tapping as long as it is comfortable (aim for 100 or so taps to start)

> Note: This type of tapping can be quite invigorating, bringing all kinds of energy to your lower abdomen (the sacral chakra or 2nd energy center). You may want to do this kind of tapping to upbeat music.

Full-body tapping is usually done with loose fists or with cupped palms. Tap the body using the side of your fist away from the thumb. You may use one fist when tapping an arm or hand or both fists when tapping other parts of the body.

- Stand or sit comfortably
- Start tapping the lower belly, using both hands while tapping on the same spot two inches below the navel; use this belly tapping as a general warm-up, continuing it until your lower belly feels warm (you can tap right, left, or both hands at the same time; I prefer loose fists to tap right, left and cupped palms to tap at the same time)
- Use one hand to tap the opposite arm, starting at the shoulder, with your arm stretched out and the palm up, tap the upper side of your arm down to the hand
- Turn your arm over and tap it coming back up from the hand to the shoulder

- Turn your arm part way, sticking your thumb straight up, and tap from your shoulder down your arm, ending at the thumb
- Raise your arm up and tap on the underside of your arm, ending at the armpit (tap the underarm vigorously as a lot of emotional tension is held here)
- Repeat this arm tapping for the other arm using your other fist
- Use both hands to tap down your legs from your hips to your feet (you can tap down on the outside of the leg and tap upward on the inside of your leg and you can tap down the front of your leg and up the back of your leg, and then change directions)
- You can use both hands to tap your chest and upper torso, upper abdomen and the rest of your body
- Tap rhythmically, firmly and vigorously; tap any area that appears to need stimulation

> Note: Full-body tapping is a general warmup exercise and can be continued as long as it is comfortable. It helps your energy flow as you are tapping along meridians. You can concentrate on one area such as your chest or all areas you can reach.

Bobbing

In my yoga classes, most people use belly tapping (both palms simultaneously or each hand alternatively with a loose fist) to warm up. Before going to belly tapping, I use bobbing. I learned this exercise at a workshop; it is the first step in a 12-step Ki Gong (energy cultivation) routine.

- Stand in a comfortable position (feet shoulder width apart and facing forward like an 11, knees slightly bent, shoulders and torso relaxed, hands loose and relaxed at your sides, pelvis tilted very slightly forward)
- Bob up and down, feeling movement at your shoulders, hands, hips, knees, and ankles
- Continue doing this for several minutes, feeling the energy from your head and torso sinking to your legs and energy coming up into your legs from the earth through the soles of your feet

The goal of this exercise is for your head and torso to become light and airy similar to balloons filled with air and for your legs to become thick with energy like tree trunks. For me (top heavy energy in the head and upper torso while thinking continually), this is a wonderful way to relieve stress, quiet my mind, and loosen up my muscles.

Doing this as part of a morning routine, half asleep, I also use this to check myself out. As I continue to bob up and down, becoming more and more relaxed, I check my body condition, starting at the head (starting at the feet also works). How does my head feel? My neck? Shoulders. Arms and hands. Chest and upper torso. Upper and lower abdomen. Hips and pelvic area. Thighs. Knees. Calves and feet. Basically, I just scan my body very slowly as I sense and acknowledge my condition while continuing to bob up and down.

If I am bobbing without scanning or acknowledging my condition, I watch the breath going in and out of my nose. When doing simple and repetitive tasks, remember to remain in the present. Observing your breathing is one way to do this. Try to remain in the present while bobbing; if thoughts come up, refocus your attention on your breath.

> *When I first started bobbing, I thought it was great and wanted everyone to do it. It was so easy with such great benefits! And then I had an accident, spraining my right knee and tearing the quadriceps on my left leg. Bobbing was impossible for several months and not comfortable for a very long time. Be aware. Know yourself and your condition. Do what feels good and right for you.*

EFT (Emotional Freedom Technique)

EFT (Emotional Freedom Technique), also known as Tapping (not to be confused with full-body tapping), is a powerful holistic healing technique shown to effectively resolve a range of issues. It is based on the combined principles of ancient Chinese acupressure and modern psychology.

EFT has become a cottage industry with a rapidly growing following. My exposure to EFT is through online videos, audios, and written material, most of which are either done or sponsored by Nick and Jessica Ortner (a brother-sister team). In addition to their books, they sponsor an annual Tapping Summit. EFT is gaining widespread acceptance and is used by Wellness advocates, life coaches, psychotherapists and related professionals to help their clients with emotional and physical issues. Studies and user self-reports are glowing about the positive effects of EFT. I always follow along when I find a video with a tapping exercise in it.

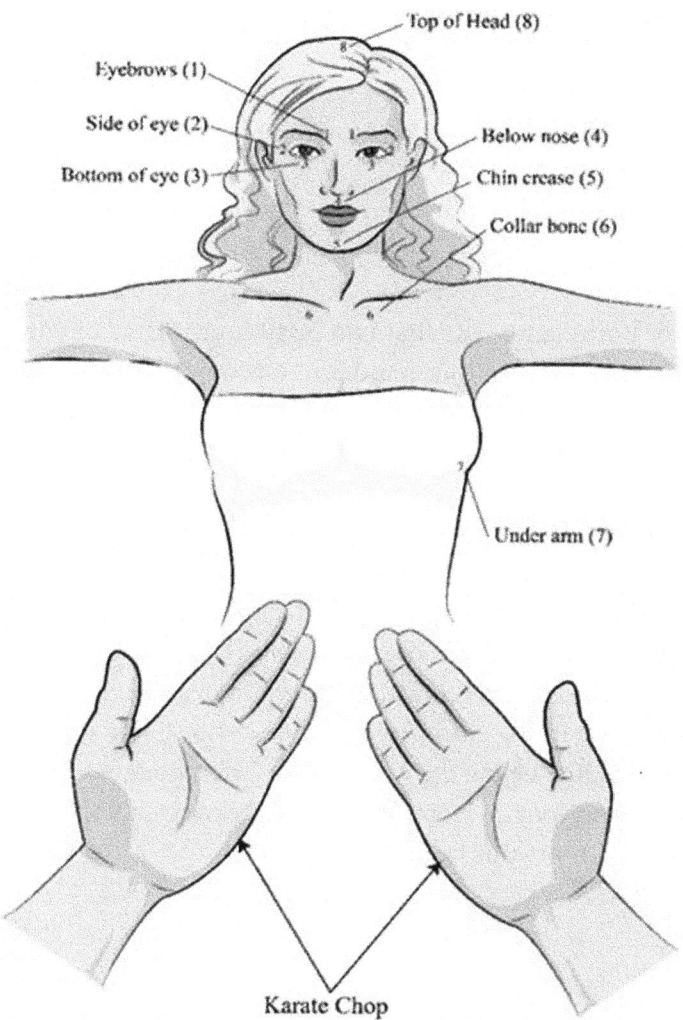

Setup

Decide on an emotional issue you want to relieve. For example, agitation over a recent argument with your spouse or friend. Rate it on a scale of 1-10 with 10 being the most severe. (If all of your emotional issues are 1 or 2, you can do something else.)

State the problem three times while tapping the karate chop (either hand; you may want to use all four fingers to tap this point) in the following format:

> Even though <the problem> I deeply love and accept myself. You may want to add adjectives for emphasis such as "I deeply love and

Yoga-Related Activities | 87

accept myself today and every day" or simplify as in "I accept myself and how I feel."

Once you finish the setup statement, go through the tapping points three times.

Tapping Points

You may use one or both hands, the first two or all four fingers of your tapping hand(s). If you are using one hand, use either hand and tap on either the left or right side. The goal of EFT is to relieve any emotional pain you may be having. Go through the tapping points three times.

1. Tap the bone ridges above the eyes where the eyebrows start from the nose area (Eyebrow = EB)
2. Tap the bone ridges on the sides of the eye (Side of the eye = SE)
3. Tap the bone ridges underneath the eyes (Under eye = UE)
4. Tap the moustache area below the nose and above the upper lip (Under nose = UN)
5. Tap the crease in the chin below the lower lip (Chin = CH)
6. Tap the area just below the collarbone (Collarbone = CB)
7. Tap the area on your side some three inches below your underarm (Underarm = UA)
8. Tap the crown of your head (Head = HD)

Procedure

1. After you state the problem three times while tapping on the karate chop, go through all of the tapping points in order one point at a time for three or more cycles, starting with the eyebrows as you state, solve, and resolve the problem. You can go from restating the problem to partial solutions to resolution while you are tapping. See the table for an example of scripting.
2. After you have done the setup 3 times, and gone through the tapping points at least 3 times, from restating the problem to full resolution, take some deep breaths and relax.
3. Re-rate your emotional issue on a scale of 1–10. If there is little or no improvement or if there is still room for improvement, you can repeat the process.

Sample EFT Script

Sample Emotional Freedom Tapping (EFT) Script			
Do the karate chop tapping continuously as you go through the setup statement 3 times. Do three rounds of detail tapping (from EB to Head) after completing the setup statement, saying the script aloud for each round.			
Karate Chop Setup	Even though I don't feel very positive right now, I accept who I am and how I feel. Even though I feel stressed right now, I choose to focus on positive emotions. Even though I'm exhausted right now, I accept all of me and how I feel.		
	Round 1	Round 2	Round 3
Eye Brow (EB)	I'm always afraid of what might happen.	I love feeling grateful.	I love feeling good.
Side-Eye (SE)	What if something bad happens to me?	I choose to feel good no matter what.	I appreciate feeling so grateful.
Under-Eye (UE)	I feel the fear every day.	I feel appreciation for being alive.	I appreciate who I am.
Under-Nose (UN)	I can feel the fear no matter what I do.	I love who I am and how I feel.	I love who I am becoming.
Chin (CH)	I don't feel safe unless I'm feeling worried.	I am grateful for my life.	I'm grateful for all my feelings.
Collar Bone (CB)	I'm afraid to let go of my fear.	I appreciate my life so much.	I appreciate the guidance I am getting.
Under Arm (UA)	I don't know how to feel any other way.	I am grateful for the clarity in my life.	I am grateful for who I am.
Head (HD)	What if I can't let go of my fear?	I love feeling so joyful.	I love feeling such joy.

This script is adapted from a Gratitude tapping session by Carol Look. In addition to being an author and psychotherapist, she uses and models EFT in her client work.

> Note: This script shows the flexibility of EFT with changes to the setup wording. The script for detail tapping goes from the problem and negativity to the solution and feeling good.

To start, tap on the karate chop point (small finger side of the hand) of one hand with the four fingertips of your other hand. State the problem situation aloud three times while continuously tapping. You can then go through the tapping points (eyebrow through the top of the head). Typically, you will go through the points at least three times with different wording and meaning each time.

In this example, after you have relieved the sensation of chronic fear in your mind and body with Meridian Tapping, you move towards more positive and appreciative thoughts and statements.

Jessica Ortner emphasizes that using your own words is the most effective scripting. For me, this is the most difficult part of tapping. What to say? In what order? Generally, the tapping script goes from what is actual/negative to changing/neutral to result/ positive. The first and second times through the tapping points may include some negativity. When questioned about reinforcing negative behavior, Nick Ortner quoted Louise Hay, "To clean a house, you first have to see the dirt."

> If possible, **view a tapping video** before you try EFT. It will be much easier to follow than the above table. This section is to introduce you to EFT and to get you curious about it. Hopefully, you will be inspired to learn more about EFT and try it. For certain physical and emotional conditions, it is simply amazing. You will be surprised by the results. See the Sources section.

Making Noise

There are several ways of making noise that helps relieve stress and keep you in the present. I call them 1-minute wonders as they only have to be done for a short period of time to be effective.

These noise makers are a great group exercise. They can also be done alone, but you will need to be away from others in order not to disturb them. Also, you do not want anyone to call the authorities while you are laughing, screaming, or otherwise making noise all by yourself.

Speaking Gibberish

This is a simple exercise with a strong underlying psychology. Briefly, you are controlled by language. You learn how to communicate and have the world imprinted on you from about two years old to six years old. Most of our beliefs are acquired early in life and are retained and reinforced throughout our lives even when they may no longer serve us. Our preconceptions may narrow and limit our world.

Speaking gibberish takes you back to before you were one year old. It is a way to stop your thinking (mind chatter) and force you to be in the present. It is a way to bring you to your zero point, to give you a few minutes without preconceptions or endless reinforcement of your beliefs, many of which no longer serve you.

- Sit or stand comfortably (if in a group, you may want to be in a circle)
- In a loud, forceful voice, start talking gibberish (you may feel silly or self-conscious, but keep with it)
- Do not use words you know or say anything with any meaning, just keep speaking gibberish

> Note: Be like a baby in a crib, chortling and talking nonsense; you can even move your arms and legs as though you were an infant.

- Speak gibberish for at least a minute (working your way up to five minutes over time)
- When you stop, take some deep breaths and check out your condition

How do you feel? Some people report feeling light-headed as though there has been a release of tension and stress or a burden has been removed from them. You may want to try talking gibberish a couple of times a day for a week or so. Is it a liberating, freeing force? Do you feel better or worse? Did you fall into the trap of starting to make sense out of your gibberish?

Laughing

Laughing is a marvelous activity that releases all kinds of tension and stress. "Laughter is good for the soul."

- Sit or stand comfortably (if in a group, you may want to be in a circle)
- Start laughing out loud (this may feel forced but keep with it)
- Laugh loud, chuckle, guffaw, belly laugh, be raucous, have fun, keep laughing

> Note: At first, this may seem really forced or fake. After laughing for a very short while, I realize how silly and ridiculous I must look and sound and start laughing for real. Laughing at myself and my situation, I laugh as loud as I can.

- Continue laughing for an entire minute
- When you stop and check out your condition, I hope you are smiling

When I first used laughter in a group setting, I asked everyone to laugh for two minutes. One woman turned to me, looking pained and said, "That's a very long time." It sure was.

Screaming

Similar to laughing aloud, screaming can be an invigorating way to release tension and stress. If you are self-conscious about speaking gibberish or laughing aloud, wait until you start screaming. This is best done in a group setting or when you are not around other people.

- Sit or stand comfortably (if in a group, you may want to be in a circle)
- Start screaming out loud (this may feel forced but keep with it)

- Scream loudly (get that throat chakra working, clear those lungs, get all of that frustration, anxiety or fear right out of you)
- Continue screaming for a couple of minutes
- When you stop, take several calming deep breaths and check out your condition

What did you do in yoga class? Oh, we had a group scream. Sure. Why not? Actually, it's a wonderful way to move blocked energy and release stress. Try it.

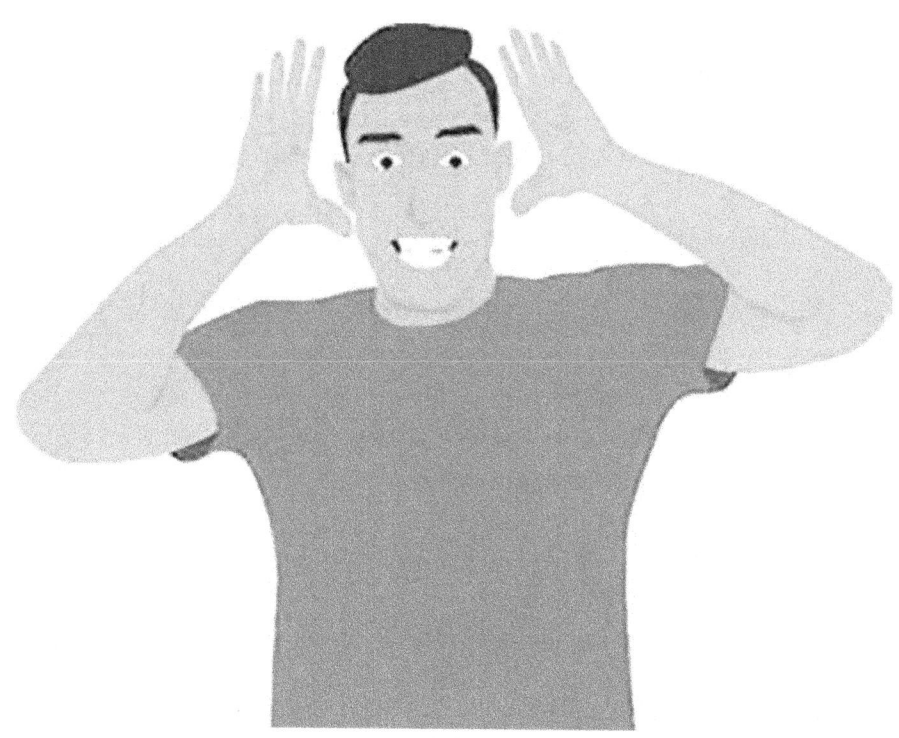

Tarzan Calling

Making noise can be combined with other yoga movements or related activities to increase its effectiveness in releasing tension and stress. For example, making a loud "Ah" sound while vigorously tapping your chest (similar to the Tarzan yell from the movies) opens your chest and lungs, as well as your heart and throat energy centers (chakras).

- Start tapping your chest using both hands (loose fists) similar to Tarzan in the movies
- While tapping, say an extended "ah" sound as loud and as long as you can
- Continue tapping vigorously and saying out loud, extended "ahhhhhhhhhhs"
- Do this for a few minutes or as long as comfortable (tap strongly, some say "pound" but be gentle with yourself; say "ah" as loud and as long as you can, pausing to take another breath)
- When you stop tapping, sweep your hands downward from your shoulders along your chest, releasing some of the accumulated energy

This is a quick, effective way to open your chest (heart and lungs). Have fun with it.

Power Posture

Ilchi Lee is the founder of Dahn Yoga. He received his enlightenment after a 21-day ordeal in the mountains in which he neither ate nor slept.

This posture is his answer to:

> *What is the simplest and most effective exercise a person can do?*

- It is referred to in Dahn Yoga as the Ilchi Li or power posture.
- Stand in a relaxed position with your feet shoulder width apart and knees slightly bent
- Stretch your hands above your head to the full extent of your arms
- Point your two index fingers straight up with your thumb and other fingers in a loose fist
- Hold this position for a minute or so, working your way up to five minutes over time

> Note: This position can also be done while lying flat on your back with your legs and arms stretched out. This may be easier on your shoulders although I prefer doing it while standing up.

This is a great way to stretch your upper back and to aid energy circulation. Sometimes, when holding this posture, I feel like a giant antenna. Either standing or lying down, I think you will enjoy this simple exercise.

Ego Eradicator

From the Kundalini Yoga tradition, Ego Eradicator helps keep the ego in check. This posture can be done while standing or sitting:

- If standing, stand with both feet flat on the floor, weight equally distributed on both feet
- If sitting on a chair, sit firmly on the chair (not all the way back) with a straight spine and feet flat on the floor
- If sitting on the floor, you can use Easy Pose, sitting in a cross-legged position with a straight spine

Follow these steps:

- Sit or stand comfortably as above
- Close your eyes and focus them at the brow point (in between the eyebrows about ¼ inch up) or keep them open looking straight ahead

> Note: If you are not used to standing up with your eyes closed or if you have issues with balance, practice this with your eyes open.

- Bring your arms out to the sides and raise them up so they form a "V" shape, holding your hands over your head
- Curl your fingers into the pads of your hands near the base of your fingers; point your thumbs out toward the sky
- Stretch up from the shoulders but don't raise them

- Do not bend your elbows or arch your spine
- Check the angle of your arms; hold them at 60 degrees
- Do Breath of Fire (inhaling and exhaling rapidly through your nose and diaphragm) for 1–3 minutes

> Note: Work your way up to 3 minutes over time; if you are unable to do a Breath of Fire, try long deep breathing.

- To end, inhale and bring your arms straight up over your head, opening your hands, with the fingers spread wide and pointing up while you touch your thumb tips together; briefly suspend your breath, then exhale

The thumbs represent the ego or persona of the individual thus the name Ego Eradicator. The thumb relates to the persona of the individual. The human quality is happiness.

Each area of the hand corresponds to a certain area of the body or brain. In this case the thumb which represents the ego or personal psyche is transformed and balanced. This exercise opens the lungs, brings the hemispheres of the brain to a state of alertness and consolidates the energy field.

Feet

Just as our face and hands are filled with nerve endings, so are the soles of our feet. The feet also contain an important energy center located just below the ball of the foot in between the second and big toes. It is located in the indentation where your footprint creates an upside-down V shape. You can stimulate this energy center by standing up straight and leaning forward very slightly (about one degree from the center of the bottom of your feet).

Toe-tapping

This is a simple, effective way to increase the circulation to your feet. It helps release emotional tension from the body, bringing energy away from your head to your lower body. When you are unable to sleep due to restlessness and a head full of worries, you can use toe-tapping to relieve your insomnia.

You can do toe-tapping while lying on your back or while sitting upright on the floor with your legs spread out in front of you. As necessary, you can sit against a wall for back support. Breathe normally, concentrating on the tapping.

- Lie on your back with your feet and legs together
- Place your arms at your sides with the palms facing upward (if you are sitting have your palms flat on the floor for balance and support)
- Flex your toes back while keeping your heels together
- Tap your big toes together, then open your feet so that your little toes touch or come close to touching the floor

Note: When first starting, concentrate on tapping your big toes. As you warm up and go more quickly it will become easier and easier to have your small toes come closer to touching the floor.

- Do the toe-tapping as rapidly as you can comfortably, starting with 100 taps (this should take a couple minutes, counting 1, 2, 3, 4, 5, 6, 7, 8, 9, <u>10</u>, then 1, 2, 3, 4, 5, 6, 7, 8, 9, <u>20</u>, etc. until you reach 100).
- To finish, continue lying on your back, breathing through your nose, eyes closed, feeling the effects of energy circulating in your body; remain resting for a couple of minutes.

Once you can tap your toes without strain or discomfort, you can add the following to aid circulation and include more of your body in the exercise:

- Gently shake your head from side to side as you continue toe-tapping
- With your palms facing upward, open and close your hands into loose fists

Note: Move your head at a pace that is comfortable for you. Open and close your hands as quickly as you can, keeping pace with your toe taps. (I do the hand opening and closing, but not the head movement as it throws off my rhythm.)

The first time I did toe-tapping for an extended period of time (300 taps or more), I stopped abruptly and felt energy surge to the top of my body. It was an enjoyable experience.

When first starting, you may feel fatigue in your hips, thighs or calves, especially if you have some energy blockages in those areas. In most cases, you can work through the blockages by doing 50-100 repetitions for several days before increasing the amount you do. If counting is too distracting, you can use a timer. Also, you can start at a slow to medium pace and work your way to a nice, rhythmic, quicker pace.

Rotating Your Feet

This is a way to stretch your feet and improve circulation. You can do this lying down or sitting on the floor with your legs stretched out in front of you.

- Lie down on the floor on your back with your hands at your sides and your legs stretched out on the floor with your feet shoulder length apart
- Rotate your feet inward, with your toes making a full circle
- Repeat this 10 times while breathing normally
- Rotate your feet outward, with your toes making a full circle
- Repeat this 10 times while breathing normally
- Rotate both feet to the right, with your toes making a full circle
- Repeat this 10 times while breathing normally
- Rotate both feet to the left, with your toes making a full circle
- Repeat this 10 times while breathing normally
- To finish, lie quietly on your back, breathing deeply, feeling the energy in your feet

Bouncing Your Knees

This is a way to loosen your hamstrings and help circulation throughout your legs. It is included here as together with toe-tapping and rotating your feet, it is good for your legs and will help them feel better. Loose, flexible hamstrings are a sign of longevity.

- Lie down on the floor on your back with your hands at your sides, knees bent, and your feet flat on the ground shoulder length apart
- Keeping the edge of your heels on the floor, bounce your knees up and down, feeling the stimulation to the backs of your knees

- Start slowly, building speed, and increasing the amount of impact on the back of your knees
- Work your way up to 100 or more repetitions; this can be used as a warmup for more vigorous stretching

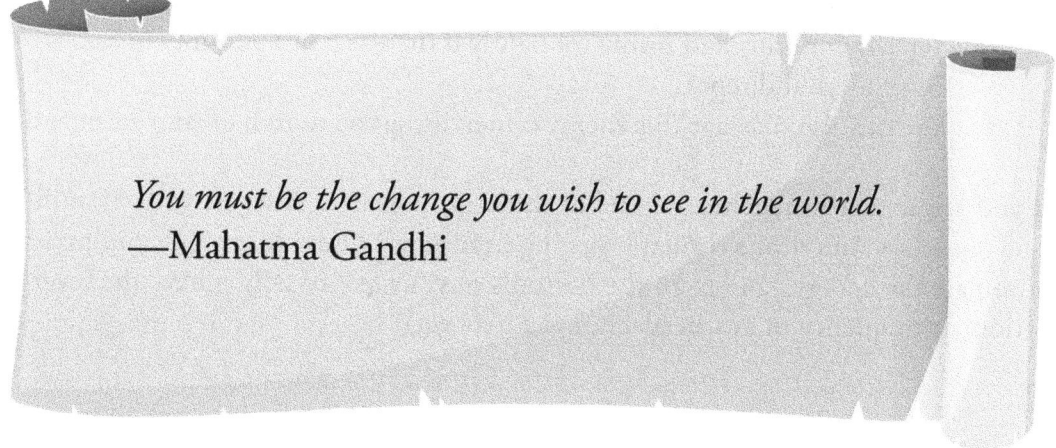

You must be the change you wish to see in the world.
—Mahatma Gandhi

Sole Tapping

This is a relatively easy way to bring energy to the bottoms of your feet. Among other things, it stimulates and helps your kidneys. It is also a way to help relieve headaches and aid clarity of mind.

> Note: If you have open sores, cuts, or swelling on the bottoms of your feet, check with your physician before doing this exercise. Do not tap too long or too hard, especially if there is pain or discomfort. Remember, you are the master of your body. Listen to it and nurture it.

You can sit on the floor with your legs extended out in front of you. As desired, you can sit against a wall or in a straight-backed chair for more support for your back. The sole of your foot has an energy center just to the inside of the ball of your foot. This is where you want to tap.

- Sit comfortably with your legs spread out in front of you
- Bend one leg over the other with the foot of your bent leg at about the level of the knee or lower thigh of your stretched out leg

- Use your hand on the same side as the crossed leg to hold your foot with the sole facing upward
- Form a light fist with your free hand and tap the bottom of the foot (just below or inside the ball of your foot) crossed over your leg with the little finger side of your fist
- Tap rhythmically and firmly (or lightly if there is pain) 30 times or so
- Switch legs and repeat
- You can also massage this energy center, using the thumb of your free hand.

Did you know that headaches are one of the most prevalent diseases with 45 million or one out of six Americans regularly getting headaches? Use sole tapping and massage to stimulate the energy centers on the bottoms of your feet to help relieve the severity, duration, or frequency of any headaches you may get.

Walking

Walking is a simple and effective way to maintain your body. Walking has long been touted as the single most effective thing you can do for arthritis. Walking is a whole-body exercise that involves some 600 muscles and 200 bones. As many wellness experts point out, we were built for movement, which is why a couch potato lifestyle can be so debilitating. Walking is one of the best ways to keep moving.

Youthful Walking

There is the Korean concept of Jangsaeng (literally, youthful longevity) walking, developed by Ilchi Lee as he recovered from a serious injury. Virtually all walking is a path to wellness. Incorporate as much of the following into your own walking as is comfortable for you. The basic principle is to keep the body symmetrical and to keep your feet parallel while walking.

- Stand straight with your shoulders relaxed and your feet parallel like the number 11, putting weight on the balls and toes of your feet
- Keep your head straight with your eyes gazing straight ahead and your chin positioned slightly inward
- Keep your chest open but not puffed out and your arms at your side in a natural position

- Keep your knees together, almost touching, and tilt your lower pelvis slightly forward
- Breathe with your lower abdomen (normal belly breathing)
- Step forward with a straight leg, letting your heel gently tap the ground
- Feel your weight transfer fully to the ball and toes of your foot
- Keep your feet parallel, stepping on either side of an imaginary line in front of the middle of your body
- Swing your arms freely as you walk and remember to smile and enjoy yourself

For this type of walking, focus on the following:

1. Step symmetrically.
2. Activate the energy center in your foot located just below the ball of your foot as you walk (tilting your pelvis slightly forward as you walk helps as does pressing on your toes as you take a step).
3. Accumulate energy in your lower abdomen by tucking your tailbone slightly upward, tightening the anus, and slightly lifting your hips.
4. Walk with joy as this is one of the best things you can do for yourself; smile and revel in your movement.
5. Engage your entire body, swinging your arms, and checking that your body parts (hip joint, back, shoulders, and arms) are in rhythm with each other.

Intestine Exercise

The second or sacral chakra (energy center) is located on the backbone by the lower abdomen. On the surface of your body, it is approximately 2 inches below the navel. This is the center of gravity when performing Tai Chi or martial arts. It is viewed as the center of creativity as well as the source of physical well-being in Dahn (energy) yoga. The Intestine Exercise stimulates this energy center and helps your overall physical well-being.

The Intestine Exercise can be done while standing, sitting or lying down. It can also be done while holding various stretches and postures. It is a wonderful way to strengthen your core, aid digestion, and accumulate energy.

- Stand with your feet flat on the floor, shoulder width apart, toes pointing forward with your weight equally distributed on both feet and your pelvis tilted slightly forward (1-2°)

- Place your thumbs on your navel with your hands forming an upside-down triangle, the ends of your fingers resting on your lower abdomen about 2 inches below your navel
- Keep your upper body relaxed and your knees slightly bent
- Pull your abdomen inward (do not push with your hands, they are just resting on your lower abdomen throughout this exercise) as though you are trying to touch your navel to your backbone
- Push your abdomen out, relaxing it completely, making it round and totally loose

> Note: To increase the effects of this exercise, tighten your buttocks as you pull your abdomen in and let them go loose as you push your abdomen out

- Continue pulling your abdomen in (squeezing) and pushing it out (releasing) and work your way up to 100 repetitions

As you do the Intestine Exercise, continue to breathe normally. The movements are <u>not</u> connected to your breath. You can do the Intestine Exercise slower or faster than you breathe. At first glance, the Intestine Exercise may appear similar to deep breathing or just normal belly breathing. It is not. Concentrate on the movements themselves, finding a comfortable pace.

If you can get into the habit of doing the Intestine Exercise daily or every other day, you will begin to see the positive effects of this exercise in a few days or at most, a couple weeks. You will certainly lose weight as you are cleansing your gut. If nothing else, you will strengthen your abdomen, tighten your buttocks and feel more energetic.

Stretching

Stretching is basic to yoga. There are many stretches you can do, from obvious body stretching to meridian stretching to organ and full-body alignment. A handful of stretches are included here. Some general principles:

- Listen to the wisdom of your body; while it is better to stretch than not stretch you do not want to injure yourself; do not force the issue and stop if there is pain

- Relax into a stretch; tensing yourself when stretching is counter-productive
- When stretching, you can stretch just a little bit more on your exhale; so, inhale, stretch and then on the exhale, stretch a little bit more
- You can breathe into a stretch, focusing on a stiff joint or muscle and releasing any tension on the exhale

Neck—Basic Stretch

Use this neck stretch to help keep your neck in alignment.

- Stand comfortably and relaxed with your feet shoulder width apart
- Slowly moving only your neck and head, stretch your neck backward, pushing your chin upward
- Bend your head to the left, trying to touch your left ear to your left shoulder
- Then bend your head to the right, trying to touch your right ear to your right shoulder
- Bring your head to an upright position and slowly turn it to the left and then to the right
- After bringing your head to the center position, slowly rotate it to the left, doing a full circle and then to the right, doing a full circle
- Repeat this until your neck begins to feel loose

Neck Stretch with Hands

You can use your hands to get a stronger neck stretch. Be sure to do this slowly without pain. Know your limits. Listen to your body.

- Clasp your hands together with your fingers intertwined and your thumbs pointing straight up
- Put your thumbs under your chin and push your head up and back
- Hold this position for a minute or so, breathing normally; release and come to center
- Wrap your right arm over your head (forearm lying on top of your head) with your right hand covering your left ear

- Pull your head gently to the right, trying to put your right ear to your right shoulder
- Hold this position for a minute or so, breathing normally; release and come to center
- Wrap your left arm over your head (forearm lying on top of your head) with your left hand covering your right ear
- Pull your head gently to the left, trying to put your left ear on to your left shoulder
- Hold this position for a minute or so, breathing normally; release and come to center
- Clasp your hands together, intertwining your fingers and thumbs
- Place the palms of your clasped hands on the back of your head near the top of it and gently pull your head down pushing your chin into your chest
- Hold this position for a minute or so, breathing normally; release and come to center

Neck Rolls

Do neck rolls in sync with your breathing. Inhale as you move your head up and around and exhale as you move it down and complete the circle. Note that on the above neck stretch you are rotating your head just to the left and right. In neck rolls you are using an up/down circle and may even brush your ears on your shoulders.

- Stand or sit comfortably
- Start with your head lowered and your chin resting on your chest
- Inhale as you roll your head to the left and upward, moving it in a circle
- Exhale as your head reaches the top and starts down
- Repeat this for 4 full circles (4 deep, slow breaths) to the left
- Continue this for 4 full head rolls to the right; be aware of your breath, inhaling as you raise your head and roll it to the right, exhaling as you lower your head and complete the circle

As with all of the movements, you can start to the left or to the right. I suggest 4 times to the left and 4 to the right. This can be more or less, depending on the condition of your body and what feels right for you.

Neck—Other

For a general relaxing of the neck, you can simply shake it side to side as in a basic "no" gesture. You can start slowly and as the neck loosens, you can continue, shaking it more vigorously. Be gentle with yourself and do not continue if there is pain. "Shake it faster than your thoughts" is a goal. Shaking tension and stress out of your head can be helpful, but do not overdo it.

Another way to loosen the neck is to simply turn your head to the left and right. Gently turn your head to the left as far as comfortable. Then to the right as far as comfortable. Do this slowly while paying attention to how your neck feels. You can start with 10-20 repetitions to each side and then do whatever feels right for you over time.

Shoulder shrugs may be good for you. Raise your shoulders up, trying to touch your ears with them. You can do about 10 of these and then check your condition. How do you feel?

I have limited range of motion in my neck and often feel tightness and stiffness. I have a tendency to do the following a couple of times a day. It seems to loosen both my neck and my shoulders.

- Inhaling, turn your head without pain as far as possible to the right and hold. Exhaling, return it to center.
- Inhaling, turn your head to the right, tilting your chin about a quarter of the way above your shoulder. Exhale as you return to center
- Inhaling, turn it to the right, chin about ¾ up, returning it to center as you exhale
- Inhaling, raise your head straight up, staring at the ceiling. Exhale as you lower your head.
- Repeat this process on your left side

Do neck rolls or gently shake your head from side by side as you finish. Doing these neck exercises helps loosen the neck and relieve tension in your shoulders. Simply turning your head left and right without forcing it to go too far is a low impact way to free up your neck.

Neck Movement—A Variation

Anat Baniel specializes in neuro-movements (small physical movements with a corresponding large change in brain functioning). In a 2015 interview with Lisa Garr, she outlined the following variation of loosening the neck by turning it side to side.

- Sit or stand comfortably
- Place the palm of one hand on your forehead (hold the hand straight, fingers extended, with the palm flat against the forehead; do <u>not</u> grip or otherwise use your hand to turn your head)
- Place the palm of your other hand on the back of the head (once again, do <u>not</u> use the hand to grip or influence the turning of your head)
- Turn your head from side to side, left to right, right to left for a few minutes
- Change your hands and repeat turning your head left and right for a few minutes

After you finish, sit quietly and notice how you feel. More relaxed? Less turmoil in your mind?

It is now "common knowledge" that movement boosts energy levels, improves your mood, promotes better sleep, and radically decreases your risk for diabetes, cancer, heart disease.

- *As little as 10 minutes of walking can lead to significant reductions in back pain.*
- *Leads to reduced frequency, intensity and duration of both headache and migraine pain.*
- *And, it has been shown to reduce joint pain in obese individuals by over 70%!*

One very large pain study with over four thousand participants, demonstrated that the greatest reductions in chronic pain were achieved by people that incorporated the greatest levels of movement into their daily lives.

Dr. Yoni Whitten support@painfixprotocol.com
www.painfixprotocol.com/

Reaching Up on Your Toes

This is good for the upper back; stretches muscles in your sides, and helps the feet and calves. Basically, you will be raising your hands over your head and rising up and down on your toes, facing forward and then to each side.

- Stand with your feet together (nearly touching), flat on the floor, facing forward
- Hold your hands waist high with the palms facing upward. Intertwine your fingers, about waist high with the palms facing upward
- Raise your hands over your head, turning them over around throat high, ending with your arms stretched straight up and your interlaced fingers facing palm upward
- With your arms raised, go up on your toes and then back down flat on the floor
- Repeat this 10 times, working your way over time to whatever number feels right for you
- Standing with your lowered feet together, facing forward, turn your upper torso from the waist as far as possible to the left with your hands still clasped over your head; try to look behind yourself but keep your feet and legs facing forward
- Go up on your toes, then back down, repeating this 10 times while twisted to the left
- Come back to center with your hands still clasped over your head
- Standing with your lowered feet together, facing forward, turn your upper torso from the waist as far as possible to the right with your hands still clasped over your head; try to look behind yourself but keep your feet and legs facing forward
- Go up on your toes, then back down, repeating this 10 times
- Come back to center, releasing and lowering your hands to your sides
- To finish, shake out your arms and legs

How do you feel? For me, twisting to the left and to the right is the most difficult part as I feel the stretch in my side. I am always careful to not overdo it.

Side Stretch

This stretch is good for your muscles all along your side and helps improve blood circulation in your abdomen.

- Stand comfortably with your feet at least shoulder length apart (you may want them wider for a better stretch)
- Place your left hand on your left leg about knee level (if comfortable)
- As you inhale, reach your right arm straight up over your ear, bending it to your left side, sliding your left hand down your leg as far as you comfortably can
- Hold this for a count of 3, keeping your body upright without leaning forward
- Exhale and return to your starting position
- Repeat this 3 times on each side

This can be vigorous. Widening your feet further apart helps the stretch.

Hip Stretch

This exercise helps open your hips and is especially good for people who sit too much.

- Lie comfortably on the floor with your legs straight
- Bend one knee, grasping your shin with both hands
- Pull the leg in toward your chest and down toward your armpit
- Inhale and hold your breath for 5 counts, then release and lower your leg as you exhale
- Repeat this 3 times on each leg

Toe Touch

Most of us have probably touched our toes (or tried to) at various times in our lives. This is a useful way to do it.

- Stand comfortably and relaxed with your feet shoulder width apart
- As you inhale slowly and deeply, raise your arms straight over your head with your hands open and your fingers pointing toward the ceiling

- As you exhale slowly, lower your arms, keeping your arms and legs straight, until you touch your toes with your fingertips
- Note: If it is too difficult to touch your toes, let your fingertips go as far as comfortable (the knee or shin is okay). If it is too easy for you to touch your toes, you can touch the floor in front of your toes or you can touch the palms of your hands to the floor.
- Return to your original position, breathing normally
- Repeat this process 10 times

After an early yoga class, during sharing, I said, "If we are as young as we are flexible, I must be 105." The woman next to me, smiled and said, "Stay with it. It took me a year but I can finally bend over and touch the floor while keeping my legs straight." I was wondering what's the big deal, when she said, "Oh, I mean I can touch the floor with the palms of my hands." She looked fit and was 72 at the time.

Rag Doll

When you are done stretching, you may want to end with this exercise. It is relaxing and a good way to release any remaining stress or tension in your body.

- Stand comfortably and relaxed with your feet shoulder width apart
- Bend over from the waist and let your head and hands dangle downward as low as comfortable
- Exert no pressure, build no tension, just let your entire body be loose and flexible like a rag doll
- As you do this, breathing normally, feel any tension or stress drain out of your hands and the top of your head
- As you continue, you may find yourself bending lower, especially on the exhale; do <u>not</u> try to do anything, just relax and release anything you do not need
- Continue until you feel really relaxed

Twist and Turn

Closely related to stretching are twisting and rotating different parts of your body. They provide a stretch as well as movement which can be beneficial.

Twist

You can start with a twist similar to the dance craze that became popular in the 1960s, then move your arms chest high and then throw your burdens over your head as you continue to twist.

- Stand comfortably and relaxed with your feet shoulder width apart and your hands held loosely waist high a few inches in front of your torso
- Twist your left hip forward and to the right as you move your right hand to the left
- Twist your right hip forward and to the left as you move your left hand to the right
- Fall into a rhythm and do this as rapidly as is comfortable, feeling your hips loosen
- Note: Music may help you get in a rhythm. Watching the twist on an old movie may help. As you let yourself go, you will enjoy the movement and freedom of "doin' the twist." Have fun.
- Raise your hands to chest level and hold them in loose fists nearly touching a few inches in front of your torso, elbows sticking out to the side
- As you twist your left hip to the right, move your hands and arms to the left; then move your hands to the right as you twist your right hip to the left
- Fall into a rhythm and do this as rapidly as is comfortable, feeling the stretch and movement in your shoulders and upper back
- Finally, as you continue to twist your hips, you can hold your hands about head high with your arms bent at the elbow
- Optionally, you can twist to the right, throwing your hands up over your head to the left and then twist your hips to the left, throwing your hands up over your head to the right

You can also do the Washing Machine version which is great for a vigorous cleansing of your abdominal area:

Stand with your feet together facing forward

- Hold your hands in loose fists around waist high
- Twist your hips right and left as you move your arms and hands in the opposite direction
- Build up to doing this as quickly and vigorously as you can
- Picture and/or imitate a washing machine, going faster and faster
- To end, stand quietly, breathing deeply, feeling the energy in your body

There are many variations to the above. For example, for a better twist you can put one foot forward in front of your body and as you twist your hips you can lean forward and backward moving your weight from one leg to the other. The goal is to loosen those muscles and help circulate your energy. Have fun with this one.

Knee Rotations

Knees are a problem for many of us. Closely related to the above twists, knee rotations help loosen the knees and prepare them for more strenuous activity.

- Stand comfortably and relaxed with your feet together
- Activate your hands, rubbing them vigorously together until they are warm, even hot
- Bend your knees slightly, keeping your feet flat on the floor
- Bend over and massage your knees, rubbing the front, sides, and back of both knees
- Relax your upper body and rest your hands on your knees, but do not put any weight on them with your hands
- Rotate your knees together in a circular motion to the right, keeping your feet flat on the floor for 10 repetitions
- Repeat the movement, circling to the left for 10 repetitions
- Rotate your knees in little circles, inside to outside, for 10 repetitions
- Repeat the movement, circling from the outside to the inside for 10 repetitions
- To finish, stand up straight and shake out your arms and legs

For a variation, stand with your feet shoulder length apart. Notice the difference as you move your feet closer or further apart.

Twist—A Qi Gong Variation

This is a low impact version of the twist that is helpful for releasing Qi energy in your body. It is a nice way to start the day. As Lee Holden says in his video showing this, "Do this to get your morning cup of 'Chee'." It is a 3-minute wakeup routine.

- Stand comfortably with your feet shoulder length apart, holding your hands at your side in loose fists
- As you twist your hips and torso slightly to the left, strike your lower abdomen with your right forearm and the base of your back with your left forearm (this is done lightly and at a moderate pace)
- As you twist your hips and torso slightly to the right, strike your lower abdomen with your left forearm and the base of your back with your right forearm
- Do this for about a minute (comfortably tapping and activating some acupressure points in your lower back and bringing energy to your abdomen)

See Figure 1 for the acupressure points stimulated by your forearms as you twist.

- As you continue twisting, bring your arms up and strike your chest where it meets your left shoulder with your right hand (knuckle side of a loose fist) and then do the same on your right side with your left hand

See Figure 2 for the acupressure points stimulated by your left and right hands.

- Do this for less than a minute
- Then as you continue twisting, slap the top of your left shoulder with the palm of your right hand and then slap the top of your right shoulder with the palm of your left hand
- Stop twisting, and begin tapping the center of your chest with the knuckle sides of your loose fists (basically tapping the sternum from your neck to its end)
- Sweep the energy downward from your chest
- Close with three deep breaths, raising your arms over your head touching your fingertips together and then lowering your arms on the exhale

Figure 1—Acupressure Points at Base of Spine

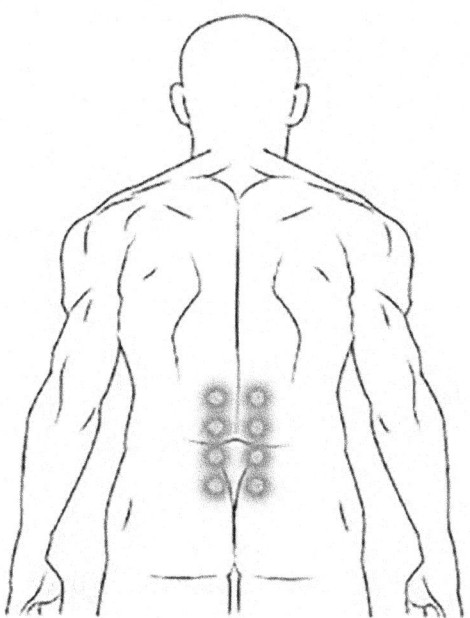

As you twist, let your forearms stimulate these lower back points.

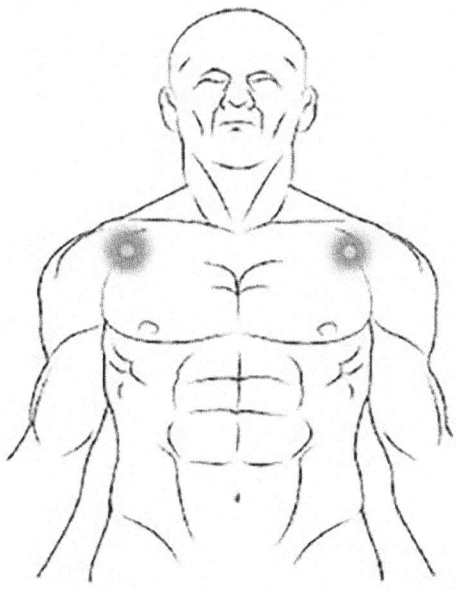

As you continue to twist, use your hands (loose fists work) to stimulate these shoulder points.

Yoga-Related Activities | 113

Summary

I think of these as yoga-related activities. Except for EFT (Emotional Freedom Technique) which uses meridian tapping, I was introduced to all of these activities during yoga classes or seminars. Many of them are used for warming up, releasing stress, and preparing the body for meditation or more strenuous physical exercises.

Body tapping and bobbing are great warmup exercises, as is the intestine exercise. You can also do them on their own. These three exercises are really helpful and among my favorites. I would suggest doing at least one of them on a regular basis. I do the intestine exercise daily.

Stretching is basic to yoga and a good way to become more limber and circulate energy to different parts of your body. Several stretches, including neck stretches, are included here.

Twisting can be an enjoyable way to circulate and release energy. With the movements similar to the dance Twist, you can do these exercises to upbeat music. Knee rotations help relax and loosen your knees.

A Gi Gong variation of the Twist shows you how to activate several acupressure points while doing a low impact twist.

The best way to use and enjoy this chapter is to skim it and do any exercises that look interesting or helpful for your condition. They are invigorating, freeing up and moving the energy in your body.

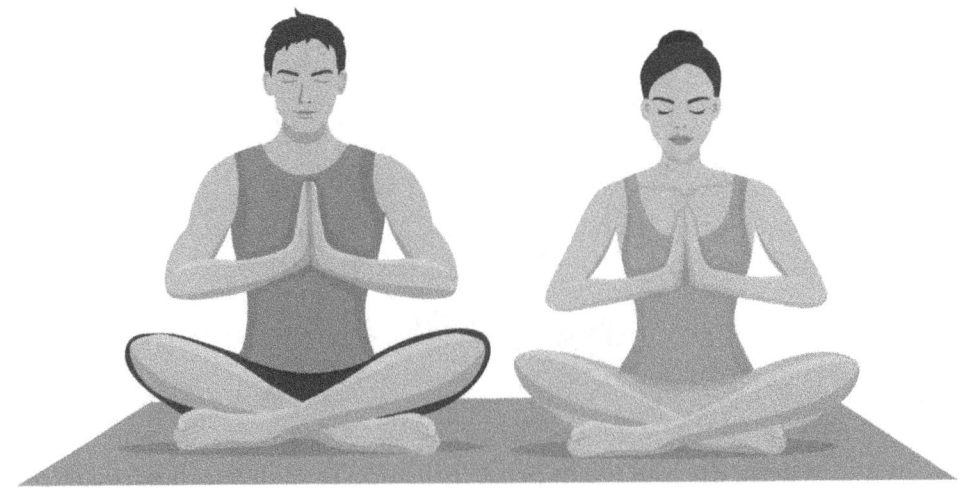

Yoga

Yoga has been defined as a discipline as well as union. As a discipline, it consists of stretches, movements, and postures performed in specific ways to achieve desired outcomes. It is a way to bring about the union of the mind, body, and spirit. It is a physical, mental, and spiritual practice or discipline that is closely intertwined with meditation. Yoga may be defined as:

- A disciplined method for attaining a goal
- A collection of techniques for strengthening the body and the mind
- A system or school of philosophy (in the Hindu system, we have a yoga of love and devotion, a yoga of knowing and so forth)

Exposed to yoga and fascinated by it in my late 20s, I practiced sporadically and basically let myself get out of shape. I then began doing yoga in my later years as a way to reclaim my body. First, I was interested in physical exercise, then rejuvenation (of mind, body, and spirit) and finally, transformation. Could this old, sick body and dull mind be transformed into an energetic, creative, productive human being? You bet it could.

I have been exposed to Hatha, Kundalini, and Dahn yoga, although I am neither a master nor an expert in any of these disciplines. Hatha yoga is physical yoga and consists of some postures with which you may be familiar. It is gaining popularity in the West and may be offered through park districts, senior centers, and self-help groups. Kundalini yoga is a way to raise the energy stored at the base of the spine. It awakens the unlimited potential that exists in everyone. Dahn (energy) yoga emphasizes brain mastery and the accumulation, circulation, and release of energy throughout the body.

This section describes some exercises from multiple sources. Yoga is intertwined with breathing and meditation. Any special breathing required by an exercise is mentioned. As with meditation, an immediate goal of yoga is to be here now, to be in the present. Both yoga and meditation have liberation as an ultimate goal.

> It is best to practice yoga with a group of like-minded individuals and an experienced teacher. Online videos and television shows are easier to follow than the written instructions in this section,
>
> I have included three routines here, two of which are from Kundalini yoga and one from Dahn yoga. They are basically good for the back.

Chair Yoga

You can perform a number of traditional yoga activities while sitting in a straight-backed chair. If you are physically challenged, this is a safe, rewarding way to receive some of the benefits of performing yoga. You can do meditation, chanting, and several exercises while sitting in a chair. If you have trouble doing traditional yoga, check to see if your neighborhood offers these classes. Chair yoga with its simple and effective exercises helped inspire this book.

What exercises and techniques can you do if you are physically challenged? The answer is a lot. You may be able to do most of the affirmations, breathing techniques, meditations, hand exercises and some of the yoga exercises in this book. Do only those that are helpful to you. Find a balance between doing too much and nothing at all.

With these yoga routines, look them over and see if any appeal to you.

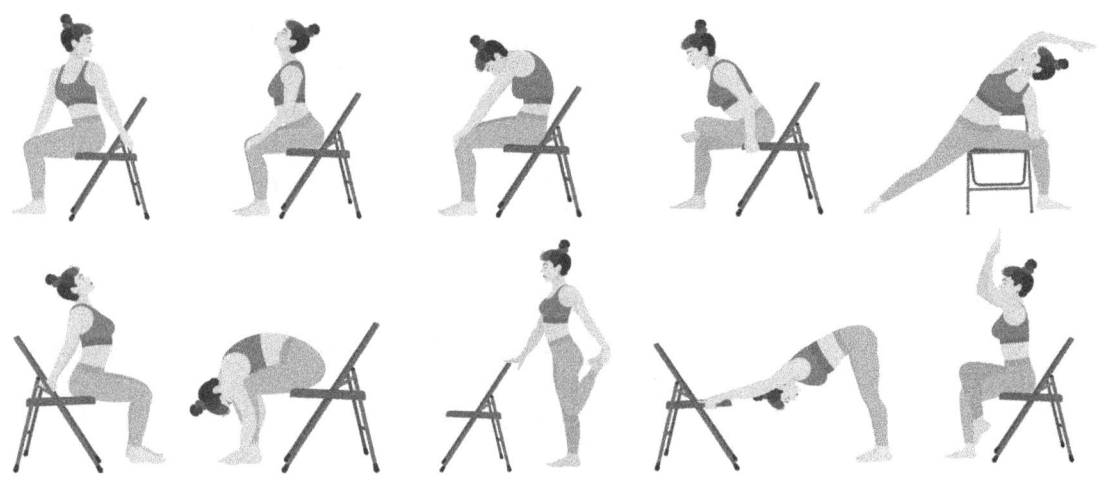

Stress Relief—Lower Back and Hip Basics

The following exercises are lower back and hip exercises to relieve tension and release stress.

> Note that there are five movements included here for Stress Relief for the lower back.

- Hip Opener
- Hip Opener (side to side)
- Pelvic Lifts
- Pelvic Tilts
- Back Press

Read over these five movements. After getting an overview, you may want to practice each one. Then start with the first one and do the entire routine.

Movement #1 – Hip Opener

Begin with this movement and continue through all five. Use these steps to raise and lower your legs while lying on your back.

- Lie on your back with your knees pressed into your chest
- Place your hands on your knees with your fingers pointing toward your toes
- Inhale as you drop your legs and feet down toward the floor
- Exhale as you bring the legs and feet back to your chest

  Note: Do not use your hands to push or pull your legs, they just ride on top. Your hips and legs do the work.

- Continue this exercise for one minute. Inhale, then exhale. Move on to #2.

Movement #2 – Hip Opener (side to side)

- Stay on your back with your knees pressed into your chest
- Bring your arms straight out to your sides. Inhale.
- Keeping your knees bent, exhale as you drop your legs and hips to one side
- Inhale as you move your legs back to center
- Exhale as you drop your legs and hips to the other side
- Inhale as you move your legs back to center

> Note: Keep your back on the ground during the movement.

- Continue this exercise for one minute
- To finish, inhale, move your legs to the center then exhale as you drop your legs down straight
- Relax and breathe normally with your legs flat on the ground while giving yourself a few moments for energy integration. Move on to #3.

Movement #3 – Pelvic Lifts

- Stay on your back and bend your knees with your feet flat on the floor
- Keep your arms at your sides, straight and parallel to your body with palms facing down
- Inhale as you tip your pelvis towards your face pressing your lower back into the floor
- Raise your bottom, lower back, mid back, and upper back as far as comfortably possible
- Exhale as you lower your upper back, mid back, lower back, bottom, and release the pelvis
- Continue this exercise for one minute, inhaling as you raise yourself up and suspending the breath as you hold the posture for a few moments
- Exhale and lower the spine very slowly. Move on to #4.

Movement #4 – Pelvic Tilts

- Stay on your back and bend your knees with your feet flat on the floor or mat
- Keep your arms at your sides, straight and parallel to your body with palms facing down. Inhale.
- Exhale as you press your lower back into the mat while tipping your pelvis towards your face.
- Inhale and release the pelvis and back.
- Continue for one minute
- To finish, inhale then exhale. Move on to #5.

Movement #5 – Back Press

- Stay on your back and bend your knees bringing them up into your chest
- Wrap your arms around your legs and gently press them into your upper torso getting as close as you comfortably can
- Take long deep breaths – inhaling and exhaling.
- Continue for one minute
- To finish, inhale then exhale as you slowly release and lower the legs and feet
- Relax on your back and breathe normally while giving yourself a few minutes for energy integration
- When done drink a glass of water!

Read over the above five movements. You can practice them one at a time and then see if you can do them as a series of movements. Listen to your body. The purpose of these movements is to relieve stress and tension in your lower back. As necessary, check with your health care professional, especially if you feel any sharp pains.

The next group of movements are for your middle and upper back. Once again, listen to your body. No pain, no gain is a myth that does not apply to yoga. Read over the movements and see if you can do them in sequence.

Upper Back Routine

One of my instructors told me to do this upper back routine daily until my mid and upper back became more flexible and stopped hurting. This routine is basically a handful of Hatha yoga postures that you may have used or you may know about. Taken together, they provide a good stretch of your back muscles and may provide you with relief if you are having back problems. Do each posture for 10 breaths; repeat the routine three times. Breathe in through your nose and exhale through your mouth.

#1: Cat-Cow

This exercise works on points along the spine, strengthens the second chakra, the lower back, and the abdomen.

- Get down on the floor on your hands and knees with your palms flat on the ground, your body relaxed and your abdomen totally relaxed (like a cow)
- Hands shoulder width apart, knees hip width apart, fingers spread wide
- As you inhale through your nose, bring your head all the way up and arch your spine
- As you exhale, round your back and let your head drop down with your back curving upward (like a cat doing a morning stretch)
- Establish a smooth routine, inhaling, head up, exhaling, head down with back rounded upward
- Continue for 10 breaths and move to #2: Sphinx

#2: Sphinx

- From the cat-cow kneeling position slide your arms forward, resting your forearms on the floor
- Stretch your legs out behind you
- Keep your head up and level, looking straight ahead (remain in this position like a Sphinx)
- Continue for 10 breaths (inhale through your nose, exhale through your mouth) and move to #3: Cobra

#3: Cobra

- From the Sphinx position, lie on your stomach with your chin on the ground, bringing your hands underneath your shoulders with the palms facing downward
- Hands shoulder width apart, shoulders down and relaxed
- Inhale, raising your head up and back; continue upwards, raising the upper portion of your body while keeping your pelvis on or as close to the ground as comfortably possible
- Remain in this position with your head back, arms straight, and your pelvis on the ground (like a Cobra that has risen to a flute)

> Note: If it is difficult to keep your arms straight, bend your elbows or put your forearms on the ground in ½ Cobra

- Continue for 10 breaths, breathing in through your nose and exhaling through your mouth (for greater effect you can tighten your buttocks on the exhale and relax them on the inhale); move to #4 Child Pose

#4: Child Pose

- From the Cobra position, come up on your knees and bend backwards, sitting on your ankles (if this is too painful do not sit all of the way back)
- Bend forward, putting your forehead on the floor and your arms stretched out over your head with your palms facing down or your arms by your sides with your palms facing up
- Remain in this position, relaxing completely (like a child asked to put his or her head down and get some rest)
- Continue for 10 breaths, breathing in through your nose and exhaling through your mouth
- Go to #1 Cat-Cow or finish

If you have completed three repetitions of this routine, lie on your back with your arms at your sides and your legs stretched out. Relax completely and notice how your body is feeling.

Wake Up and Move in the Morning

This set can help get you going in the morning. Use it to warm up, renew your energy, and give yourself a clearer perspective to help you start your day. Do all of these movements while standing.

You can do any of these movements during the day as well. Practice these movements as a set, select a few, or use them individually. Yogi March and Cross Crawls have some similarities. A general guideline is to choose one or the other when doing this set. If you are feeling you would like to do more, you can do both using less time for each. Another option is to do Yogi March and then do Cross Crawls the next day for some variety.

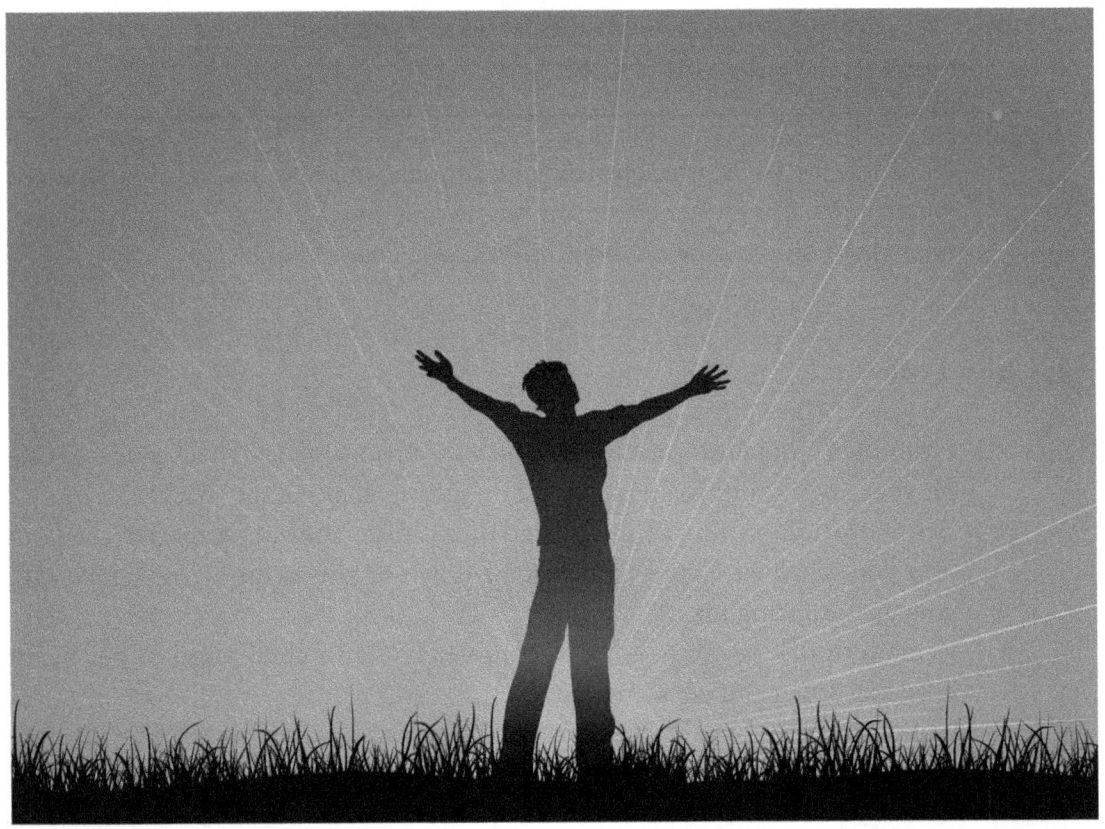

Breath—Long Deep Breathing

Relax yourself by doing some deep breathing.

- Relax your neck and shoulders as you inhale slowly, long, and deeply into the abdomen
- Allow your abdomen to fill and expand as your chest rises to fully receive the complete breath
- As you start to exhale, let your chest relax before pulling your navel back towards your spine, expelling all of the air
- Continue this pattern of inhaling and exhaling, placing your palms on your abdomen and feeling your belly expand on the inhale and contract on the exhale
- Continue this deep breathing for five breaths
- If sitting, stand up; if standing, stretch comfortably
- Take five more deep breaths

Yogi March

The Yogi March provides a nice warm up for the whole body. As you begin, move at a slow pace until you find your rhythm. You will be raising your hands from ear level to raising them straight overhead while raising one of your legs, bending it at the knee. You will alternate legs and coordinate your movements with your breathing.

- Stand with your feet flat on the floor, shoulder width apart, toes pointing forward with your weight equally distributed on both feet
- Begin raising and lowering your legs bending at the knee
- Raise your arms up and down, arms bent at your sides with your hands at ear level in the down position and then over your head and straight up in the up position
- Keep your hands in Gyan Mudra, pressing the thumb and index fingers together at the tip—the pad or fleshy part, not the fingernails
- Inhale, raising your arms up with both feet flat on the floor
- Exhale, lowering your arms, and raising one leg, bending at the knee
- Inhale, raising your arms up with both feet flat on the floor
- Exhale, lowering your arms and raising the other leg, bending at the knee

> Note: You can do this movement slow, medium, or fast. Begin slowly; once you find your pace you can pick it up as desired.

- Continue for 1–2 minutes
- To end: inhale, exhale, and release

Cross Crawls

Cross Crawls is another great movement to do in the morning. It warms up the body as well as balancing the right and left hemispheres of the brain. This movement has some similarities to swimming when using the crawl. As with the Yogi March, begin this movement at a slow pace until you find your own rhythm.

- Stand with your feet flat on the floor, shoulder width apart, toes pointing forward with your weight equally distributed on both feet
- Keep your arms straight, down at your sides, fingers pointing down with the palms facing in toward each other
- Start with a slow pace and work your way up to a comfortable, medium pace
- Inhale, raising your right arm and left knee at the same time (As you raise your right arm up, begin bending it at the elbow; as you continue raising your arm, straighten it until it's all the way up, with your fingers pointing toward the ceiling and your palm facing in)
- Exhale, lowering your right arm and left knee at the same time (As you lower your right arm, begin bending your elbow; when you are about halfway begin straightening your arm as you lower it down, with your fingers pointing toward the floor and your palm facing in)
- As you begin lowering your right arm begin raising your left arm at the same time while raising your right knee
- Follow the same pattern on the opposite side
- Continue to do this movement while alternating sides
- As one foot touches the ground, raise the other foot
- Throughout the movement hands are open facing in towards each other
- Hands pass each other so you have both arms moving at the same time
- Keep your spine in neutral alignment and your core stable

- You can do this movement at a slow or medium pace
- Continue for 1-2 minutes
- To end: inhale, exhale, and release

Reverse Cross Crawls

- This movement is the opposite of Cross Crawls. It is good for your memory.
- Stand with your feet flat on the floor, shoulder width apart, toes pointing forward with your weight equally distributed on both feet
- Start this movement with your arms straight at your sides
- Inhale, continuing to face forward
- Exhale, bending your left leg as you raise your left foot behind you
- Tap your left heel or ankle with your right hand
- Inhale, lowering your left leg
- Exhale, bending your right leg as you raise your right foot behind you
- Tap your right heel or ankle with your left hand
- Inhale, lowering your right leg
- Continue for 1-2 minutes, alternating legs as above (left, right, left…)
- To end: inhale, exhale, and release

Front Stretch

This movement is a good way to stretch the lower back and hamstrings. It is a slow easy movement so take your time.

- Stand with your feet flat on the floor, shoulder width apart, toes pointing forward with your weight equally distributed on both feet
- Begin with your arms at your sides
- Inhale, raising your arms all the way up, keeping them straight, with palms open and fingers pointed towards the ceiling
- Hook your thumbs together
- Exhale, while gently folding forward, bending at the waist, head aligned with torso

- Stretch your arms out as you continue to lower them
- Continue all the way down until you reach your shins, feet, or the floor, depending on how far you can stretch
- Inhale, coming back up as your stretch your arms out until you are back up and your hands are stretching all the way up towards the ceiling
- Continue for 1-2 minutes
- To end: inhale, exhale, and release

Squat and Pull

The squat strengthens the thighs and buttocks. The pull works on the biceps.

- Stand with your feet flat on the floor, shoulder width apart, toes pointing forward with your weight equally distributed on both feet
- Inhale. Bring your arms straight in front of you, parallel to the ground with the palms facing up
- Exhale. Squat down half way as you bend your knees
- At the same time, close your hands as you pull your arms back bending them at the elbows
- When squatting down, your hips or buttocks should not go below your knees; this is a half way squat for your thighs, buttocks, and arms
- Inhale. Come back up as you straighten the legs and bring the arms forward and straight in front, opening up the hands
- Continue the movement up and down for 1-2 minutes
- Note: If you are not use to doing squats, start with one minute and work your way up
- To end: inhale, exhale, and release

Archer Pose

This is a good posture for courage, nervous system strength, balance, and grounding. It opens and strengthens the hips, and puts pressure on the thigh bone, balancing calcium, magnesium, potassium, and sodium.

- Come to a standing position, facing forward
- Bring your left leg out in front of you. Align your right leg with your front leg keeping it in place with your right foot facing out to the right side. Legs are about 2-3 feet apart.
- Bend your left knee so you cannot see your toes without leaning forward
- Keep your torso straight, do not arch the back, hold your right leg straight
- Put 70% of your weight on your front foot
- Draw the navel back towards the spine which strengthens the abdominals and lengthens the lower back
- Bring your left arm up and straight out in front of you parallel to the ground
- Pull your right arm all the way back as if you had a bow and arrow, curl your fingers into the pads of your hands with thumbs pointing up
- As you gaze out over the top of your left thumb find a focal point straight ahead in front of you and hold that focus
- Continue this movement for 1-3 minutes while practicing long, deep breathing
- Repeat these steps using your other side (right foot in front, left arm back)

Summary

Yoga can be viewed as a discipline or as the union of mind, body, and spirit.

Chair yoga is a way to experience some of the benefits of doing yoga while doing exercises in a less physically challenging manner.

The Stress Relief routine consists of five exercises. After trying each one, see if you can do them in order as a routine. The Upper Back routine consists of four Hatha (physical) yoga exercises. This was a routine I was assigned to do to help my middle and upper back. The four poses (Cat-Cow, Sphinx, Cobra, and Child's Pose) are traditional physical yoga postures (asanas).

The Wake Up in the Morning consists of several procedures that can be done separately or as a set.

I believe that yoga is best learned through an instructor and is best done in a group setting with like-minded people. As such, I view the yoga section as a reference tool, to help you see the variety of movements and also, to see what is available. Also, if you go to a yoga class or watch a video, these steps may help to reinforce what you learned and help you to perform the exercises on your own at home.

Yoga is a wonderful thing. Try some of the warm-up exercises (toe-tapping, bobbing, intestinal exercise), and exercises such as the Tarzan yell, stretches and twists. Do the routines in this section as you gain more expertise.

Have fun. Be positive. Live well.

Sources and Additional Information

> Nothing in this book should be considered an endorsement or advertisement for any product or service for anything or anyone. These are some of the activities and information which have helped me in my journey.

First of all, many thanks to Jan, a long-time friend, who provided the content for the kundalini exercises and information in this book. She is a kundalini yoga instructor in central Texas.

As I began writing, I realized that I had stacks of notes but little or no references (I had not planned to write a book). This section is the result of that lack. I spent my time trying to explain and document things important to me without giving credit to the source. Since most of the content of this book is well-known and accepted in certain circles, I hope this is sufficient. Except for my personal experiences, I am not the source of any of the knowledge in this work and have noted sources as available.

Getting Started

This is common or widespread knowledge echoed by many sources.

The Kung Fu Panda quote is from the movie and was quoted as hearsay in Deepak Chopra's *Seven Laws of Spiritual Success*. I do not know the original source, but enjoyed quoting a cartoon character. The ½ page on living in the present may be the most important thing in this book.

I learned about 21 days from taking 21-day meditation classes through Copra.com and from workshop follow-ups (repeat this exercise for the next 21 days). Try doing (or not doing) just about anything for 21 days at approximately the same time and you will see habits take root.

The soles of your feet, palms of your hand, and your face are filled with nerve endings. If possible, exercise barefoot or with nonslip socks to take full advantage of the nerve endings in the bottoms of your feet.

Counting in this way (1,2,3,4,5,6,7,8,9,10, 1,2,3,4,5,6,7,8,9,20…) is how it was done in my Dahn Yoga classes and is a good way to keep track of a large number of repetitions.

Scanning (checking your condition and how you feel) is an effective way to stay in the present and become self-aware.

Energy

This section describes the energy body and the concept of Chakras, both of which are key to the practice of yoga and meditation.

The quote from Jean Huston is from an email describing one of her seminars as reported by Melissa Kruz (see JeanHuston.org).

The "energy goes where attention goes" and the description of the energy body are from Dahn Yoga training and the literature.

The chart on the seven major chakras and corresponding detail are abstracted and adapted from *Wheels of Life* by Anodea Judith, Ph.D.

A picture of energy centers was sent to me by one of my Dahn Yoga instructors when I was leading Energy Meditation Circles and revised for this work.

Although details and language differ, the wisdom religions would basically agree that our energy body is composed of chakras, meridians, and acupuncture/acupressure points.

The life force that flows in us (Ki, Qi, Chi, or Prana) is germane to both meditation and yoga. As you become more aware of, and sensitive to the life force within you, as you learn to cultivate it, you can improve your health and well-being by accumulating, circulating, and releasing this energy.

Your energy goes where your attention goes. Nice words to live by.

Self

Variations of these self-examination questions are used extensively throughout the Wellness literature. I learned and practiced the questions presented here at Dahn yoga.

Slomo Shoham's anecdote about the Russian mystic is from a series of short videos done by him through Humanity's team (humanitystream.org) in connection with his *Future Intelligence* program.

The idea of preconceptions is an important one. Our personalities are basically formed by the time we are six years old and we have all kinds of ideas and beliefs which no longer serve us. The "I am solid" and "I am separate" preconceptions are presented here as wakeup calls. This entire section is based on my background in psychology, Dahn yoga, and the Wellness literature.

The Four Steps to Forgiveness is a favorite of mine, also learned through Dahn yoga. In addition to using this to ask others to forgive you, you may want to use these steps to forgive yourself.

Thinking

I used 12,000 to 60,000 thoughts from Nick Ortner; other sources say 60-80,000. Either way, we have many thoughts with most of them negative and repetitive.

Affirmations have been with us for a while and these concepts are widespread.

Mirror Work: Adapted from 4 videos presented by Robert Holden as a free introduction through Hay House (http://www.hayhouse.com/). Louise Hay is the maven of mirror work and Hay House has at least one website devoted to affirmations. You can check them out at the following website: http://www.louisehay.com/affirmations.

There are so many great sources for affirmations. These are a couple from an online meditation for weight loss conducted by Jon Gabriel (of the 226 lb. weight loss) and Carol Look:

- I radiate health and vitality, I naturally release excess weight
- I radiate healing light, I am life force vitality
- I have power, power to create my ideal body and ideal life

You may want to check out thegabrielmethod.com.

The Secret (2006), and the different video versions by the same name, are the basis for the popularization of the law of attraction. As an energy being, what you get is what you give. Like attracts like. If you want to hang around happy, vibrant people, then be a happy, vibrant person.

The reference to Silva is to the Silva Method. I took the original course (then called Silva Mind Control) in 1971 and have taken a recent course through Mind Valley, a recommended resource for training materials. Founded by Jose Silva, the Silva Method is now run by his daughter, Laura.

I receive daily affirmations for chakra healing and balancing from Angela Carter at Bioenergetics.com. I really enjoy them. Sitting quietly, I say the affirmation for the day out loud seven times.

Breathing

This is from several sources and personal experience gathered over the years. I usually start a meditation class with the Mindfulness exercise on watching your breath, especially if the participants are new. The Calming, Energizing Breath is adapted from a free video by Lee Holden distributed through Mind Valley (mindvalley.com).

The Healing Breath is from Dr. Andrew Weil and the Buddhist breath, also called 4-part breathing, is from several sources. The Long Deep Breathing and Breath of Fire are from the Kundalini tradition.

Focusing on the breath going in and out of your nose is something I have been doing for decades, probably first learned from Ram Dass (Richard Alpert) of LSD notoriety.

It is a straightforward way to begin meditating. Focusing on your breath is generally considered to be one of the most effective ways to meditate.

Meditation

The benefits of meditation are legion. Even if you just sit quietly for five minutes a day watching your breath go in and out of your nose, it will be good for you.

Breathing slowly and deeply, together with focus on an object or sound (mantra) are key to meditation.

Most of us have endless chatter in our brain and meditation is one way to quiet and calm yourself.

The mantras are basically from online 21-day meditations by Deepak Chopra (discusses the centering thought and introduces the mantra) with the rest of the time spent meditating on the mantra. They are presented through the Chopra Center (chopracenter@chopra.com).

The online services I have used have been reputable, mostly free, and you can subscribe or unsubscribe easily.

I first learned about brain waves in a Silva Mind Control course in 1971. More recently, I have taken a Silva Method course through Mind Valley. Created by Jose Silva, the Silva Method is now run by his daughter, Laura.

One way to look at brain waves and meditation is to think of an iceberg. Our conscious mind is the very top tip of the iceberg and our subconscious mind is the bulk of the iceberg. While they say about 10% of an iceberg is visible above the water, the difference between our conscious and subconscious minds is much greater. Some say the subconscious mind is 1,000 times more powerful than the conscious mind. This could easily be a much greater number.

Meditation (relaxation, breathing, focus) enables us to tap into our subconscious mind as our brain waves become slower. In effect, we can be in a deeper state of mind while still conscious. By developing our observer mind we can watch this incredible panorama with equanimity.

Meditation is much more than tapping into the subconscious mind, which is why I included the quotes from the mystic Osho from *Meditation for Busy People*. Check out Osho's website (Osho.com). There is also an online newsletter.

Hands

Warming up the hands is from Dahn yoga classes, rubbing the knuckles is from Lee Holden. Palming is from a workshop on improving eyesight taken years ago. The Hand Crease pressure point is from a Lee Holden video and the Pledge of Allegiance is from an online interview by Lisa Garr.

For more information about mudras (hand gestures) refer to *Mudras, Yoga in Your Hands* by Gertrud Hurschi.

Her book has a thorough explanation of mudras including their history. She offers great illustrations and a complete description on how to do each hand gesture. She has also included visualizations and affirmations.

You may also want to see *Healing Mudras, Yoga in Your Hands* by Sabrina Mesko, which was my introduction to finding out what a mudra is.

Several of these mudras, including the Joint Mudra are from my Kundalini collaborator.

Yoga-Related Activities

Tapping and bobbing are fun and easy. The intestine exercise helps you to clear clutter and toxins from your intestines. I use an exercise video from Dahn yoga, in which the instructor states that if you do the intestine exercise for five minutes a day, you are guaranteed to lose weight. It works.

The stretches and neck exercises were all learned in yoga classes.

EFT (Emotional Freedom Tapping) is a simple, effective way to relieve physical pain and emotional duress. I strongly recommend EFT to anyone I know. The picture of the tapping points is a revised picture taken from p. 12 of the Tapping Solution eBook and the sample EFT script was adapted from pages 20-21. See http://www.// thetappingsolution. com for all kinds of information and sample videos on EFT.

Making Noise is a favorite of mine. I have basically done these in a group setting. If you are doing them alone, make sure that anyone WHO can hear you knows you are okay (especially the screaming, although laughing, talking gibberish and the Tarzan yell can also cause alarm when you are doing them by yourself).

Yoga

Yoga is a wonderful way to gain fitness as well as union of mind, body and spirit. Movements can range from very involved and difficult to simple and easy. This section contains mostly low impact activities that you may be able to do depending on your condition. As with meditation, it would be good to get into the habit of doing some exercise each day such as youthful walking.

Some years ago, Jan had an aging uncle (then in his late 80s) and led him and a few of us in a chair yoga session. It's nice to be able to do so many beneficial things while sitting in a chair. This experience planted some of the seeds that eventually turned into this book. If your condition warrants it, you may want to check local resources (park district, YMCA, YWCA, yoga center, seniors club, etc.) to see if they offer chair yoga.

Humans were built for movement so being a couch potato will only increase physical difficulties, especially as you age. I love a quote from Dr. Christiane Northup, "Getting older is inevitable, aging is optional." Keeping a clear head (through meditation) and a fit body (through yoga and related activities) is a wonderful way to enjoy many quality years, especially if you live in the present and are mindful of your thoughts, feelings, and actions.

The exercises have been adapted from Hatha yoga, Dahn yoga, and the Kundalini tradition. See if any appeal to you. The first two groups (Stress Relief and Upper Back) should be done as a set as possible.

Books

Byrne, Rhonda. *The Secret*. Hillsboro, Oregon: Beyond Words Publishing, 2006.
> The book and related videos resulted in the popularization of the law of attraction. When I first saw the video, I summed it up in three words: "Thoughts become things."

Chopra, Deepak. *The Seven Spiritual Laws of Success: A Practical Guide to the Fulfillment of your Dreams*. San Rafael, California: 1994.
> Based on Creating Affluence: Wealth Consciousness in the Field of All Possibilities, this is a classic and one of my favorites.

Gach, Michael Reed with Marco, Carolyn. *Acu-Yoga, The Acupressure Stress Management Book*. Tokyo and New York: Japan Publications, Inc., 1981.

Hanson, Rick. *Buddha's Brain*. 1981.

Hurschi, Gertrud. *Mudras: Yoga in Your Hands.*
    This book has a thorough explanation of mudras including its history. She offers great illustrations and a complete description on how to do each one. She has also included visualizations and affirmations.

Khalsa, Shakta Kaur. *Kundalini Yoga.*
    This is one of the most comprehensive Kundalini Yoga books around. It has the basics of warm-ups, breath, mudras, lots of great kriyas, meditations, and information about the chakras, and 10 bodies. It is well-illustrated and is very easy to understand as Shakta Kaur is very down to earth.

Lee, Ilchi. Healing Chakras: *Awaken Your Body's Energy System to Complete Health, Happiness, and Peace.* Sedona, Arizona: Best Life Media, 2005, 2009.
    Background and techniques to heal chakras; comes with a meditation CD.

Lee, Ilchi and Jessie Jones. *In Full Bloom: A Brain Education Guide for Successful Aging.* Sedona, Arizona: Best Life Media, 2008.
    Background to brain education with illustrated exercises.

Lee, Ilchi. Human Technology: *A Toolkit for Authentic Living. Sedona, Arizona: Healing Society,* 2005.
    An introduction to basic concepts of self-healing by Ilchi Lee, the founder of Dahn Yoga.

Mesko, Sabrina. *Healing Mudras: Yoga for Your Hands.* New York: Ballantine, 2000.
    A straightforward description of popular mudras with illustrations and related mantras.

Web Sites

These were used directly or indirectly in this book and may start with http:// or http://www. I have used each one more than once and believe them to be stable and safe.

Web Sites

101powerfulaffirmations.com	I registered, downloaded the free eBook and unsubscribed which works with many free online samples. In some cases, you may want to stay on the mailing list.
Bodynbrain.com	Dahn Yoga. You can view this as an extension of the Body and Brain yoga and workshop classes.
Changeyourenergy.com	Dahn Yoga. Per Ilchi Lee, "*Change Your Energy. Reinvent Your Life. Transform the World.*"
Chopra.com	Virtually every word from Deepak Chopra resonates with me. Check out the 21-week meditations, periodically offered free with an option to buy for continued use.
Christywhitman.com	Christy has a Monday morning video, newsletter, and more. Not used directly, she is upbeat with good information.
Devapremalmiten.com	Some great music and chanting meditations.
EckhartTollenow.com	The master of NOW. He and Kim Eng have some nice videos that will help you stay in the present (presence). He sees a new awakening of consciousness coming.
Hayhouse.com	As with Chopra, you can get lost in the amount of really good information. Also sponsors summits.
Humanitystream.org	Online transformational courses. "*Elevating humanity, one person at a time.*"
Ilchi.com	Dahn Yoga. This site is centered around Ilchi Li, his books and teachings. "*To live an authentic life, you must take back your brain.*"
JeanHouston.com	Decades of wisdom.

Juanpablobarahona.com	Juan Pablo and his partner, Regan Hillyer, are exceptional people. I really enjoy their online meditations.
Mindmoviesmail.com	Mind movies (affirmation videos) that you can watch and create.
Mindvalley.com	All kinds of really nice material. Some free meditations, words of wisdom, master classes, and all kinds of courses. My source for Silva and Lee Holden (Qi Gong).
Soundstrue.com	Online training, events, podcasts and more. I like their motto, "Waking up the world."
Theawareshow.com	Lisa Garr is a wonderful interviewer, hosts summits and more. I used two of her interviews in this work.
Thegabrielmethod.com	He of the 226 lb. weight loss. Although not used directly, an online meditation hosted by Jon Gabriel and Carol Look on weight loss is really powerful.
Theshiftnetwork.com	Transformational education, media and events. Some great teachers and content.
Thetappingsolution.com	A must-see if you are new to EFT (Emotional Freedom Technique). Videos, eBooks, and more. This web site is a good way to understand and use EFT.
Youryearofmiracles.com	Marci Smirnoff, Lisa Garr, and Dr. Sue Morter provide positive information about manifestation.

Sing like no one's listening, love like you've never been hurt, dance like nobody's watching, and live like it is heaven on earth.
—Mark Twain

Going Forward

Some suggestions for you on your road to wellness.

Be Positive

Per Louise Hay, *"Every thought we think and word we speak affects our future. If you can change your thinking, you can change your life."* Become aware of any negative chatter in your brain and replace it with positive affirmations. You will be happier.

Breathe Well

How you breathe affects your thoughts, emotions, and physical condition. Breathing well is perhaps the most important thing you can do for your health. If you have COPD, asthma or other adverse conditions, please check with your health care provider to see if there are breathing techniques or exercises you can do to help your condition.

This book has emphasized breathing through your nose, abdominal breathing, and taking deep, regular breaths. It has also provided several breathing exercises.

Be Mindful

Live in the present. It is all we really have. Be aware of your thoughts, emotions, body sensations, and environment NOW. If anything in this book helps you "be here now," reading it has been a worthwhile endeavor.

Meditate

Get in the habit of meditating each day if only for a few minutes. Meditation is the most powerful activity that I have encountered. While many life coaches recommend ½ hour in the morning and a ½ hour at night, even 5–10 minutes can be beneficial, especially if done daily. Relax and let go of any tension you may have. Release the chatter in your brain and stress in your body. Focus. Breathe. Meditate.

Keep Moving

We were built for movement. Youthful walking and other low impact exercises are beneficial for most of us. Bobbing, tapping, and stretching are all conducive to health and well-being. Do what you can. Do an activity which makes you feel better. A really good yoga session can be blissful as you free the energy channels in your body.

May you be healthy, happy and live well.

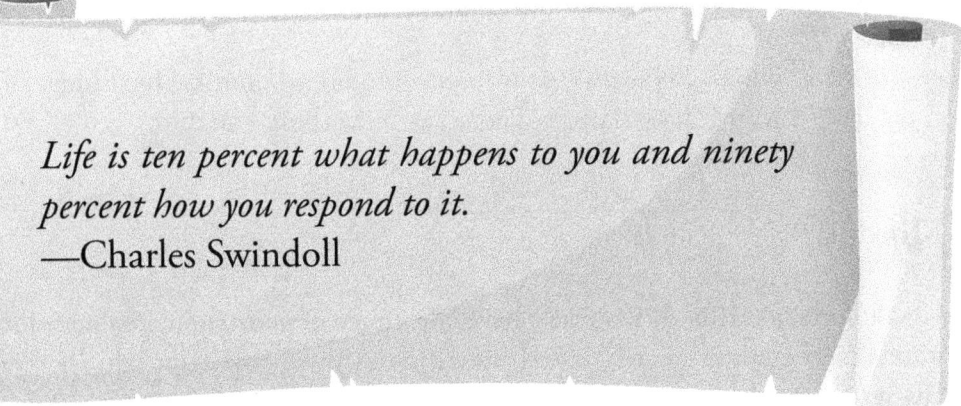

Life is ten percent what happens to you and ninety percent how you respond to it.
—Charles Swindoll

Acknowledgements

Many thanks to Jan, a long-time friend, who is also married to one of my best friends. She is a Kundalini yoga instructor living in Texas Hill Country in central Texas. Among other things, she introduced me to chair yoga and conducted some nice yoga sessions I was able to attend. She is the source for the Kundalini content (any errors are mine). She also did some editing and showed me some breathing techniques and specific activities such as Ego Eradicator and the Joint Mudra which proved useful.

Many thanks to Lorie Jones and the entire production team. They did a good job in a tight time frame. Special thanks to Aira Summers, whose support and encouragement prompted me to try one more time. Both she and Jim Addison have provided advice, encouragement and support that is truly appreciated.

I am very grateful to so many, including all of the wonderful wellness experts who are referenced in this book. Thank you all.

www.ingramcontent.com/pod-product-compliance
Lightning Source LLC
Chambersburg PA
CBHW080520030426
42337CB00023B/4574